Pediatrics

Notice

Medicine is an ever-changing science. As new research and clinical experience broaden our knowledge, changes in treatment and drug therapy are required. The editors and the publisher of this work have checked with sources believed to be reliable in their efforts to provide drug dosage schedules that are complete and in accord with the standards accepted at the time of publication. However, readers are advised to check the product information sheet included in the package of each drug they plan to administer to be certain that the information contained in these schedules is accurate and that changes have not been made in the recommended dose or in the contraindications for administration. This recommendation is of particular importance in connection with new or infrequently used drugs.

Pediatrics:

PreTest® Self-Assessment and Review
Third Edition

Edited by

Richard P. Lipman M.D., F.A.A.P.
Associate Clinical Professor of Pediatrics
Tufts University School of Medicine
Boston, Massachusetts

Senior Attending Physician
Former Chief of Medicine
North Shore Children's Hospital
Salem, Massachusetts

McGraw-Hill Book Company
Health Professions Division
PreTest Series

New York   St. Louis   San Francisco
Auckland   Bogotá   Guatemala   Hamburg
Johannesburg   Lisbon   London   Madrid
Mexico   Montreal   New Delhi   Panama
Paris   San Juan   São Paulo   Singapore
Sydney   Tokyo   Toronto

Library of Congress Cataloging in Publication Data
Main entry under title:

Pediatrics: PreTest self-assessment and review.

    Bibliography: p.
    1. Pediatrics—Examinations, questions, etc.
I. Lipman, Richard P. [DNLM: 1. Pediatrics—examination
questions. WS 18 P371]
RJ48.2.P42   1985   618.92'00076   84-12611
ISBN 0-07-051006-7 (pbk.)

34567890 HULHUL 89876

ISBN 0-07-051006-7

This book was set in English Times (Times Roman) by Allen Wayne Communica-
tions, Inc.; the editors were Beth Ann Kaufman and Irene Curran; the production
supervisor was Avé McCracken.

The Hull Printing Co., Inc. was printer and binder.

Contents

List of Contributors

Harvey L. Chernoff, M.D.
Associate Professor of Pediatrics
Tufts University School of Medicine
Senior Pediatric Cardiologist
New England Pediatric Cardiologist
New England Medical Center Hospital
(Boston Floating Hospital for Infants
  and Children)
Boston, Massachusetts

Jerome S. Haller, M.D.
Professor of Clinical Neurology
Clinical Professor of Pediatrics
Department of Psychiatry & Neurology
Tulane University School of Medicine
New Orleans, Louisiana

Julie R. Ingelfinger, M.D.
Assistant Professor of Pediatrics
Harvard Medical School
Associate in Medicine
The Children's Hospital
Boston, Massachusetts

Joseph L. Kennedy, Jr., M.D., F.A.A.P.
Associate Professor of Pediatrics
Tufts University School of Medicine
Director of Nurseries
St. Margaret's Hospital for Women
Attending Neonatologist
New England Medical Center Hospital
(Boston Floating Hospital for Infants
  and Children)
Boston, Massachusetts

Richard P. Lipman, M.D., F.A.A.P.
Associate Clinical Professor of
  Pediatrics
Tufts University School of Medicine
Boston, Massachusetts
Senior Attending Physician
Former Chief of Medicine
North Shore Children's Hospital
Salem, Massachusetts

Cody Meissner, M.D., F.A.A.P.
Assistant Professor of Pediatrics
Tufts University School of Medicine
Attending Physician in Infectious
  Disease
New England Medical Center
Boston, Massachusetts
Medical Director, Immunoserology
  Laboratory
New England Medical Center

William F. Rowley, Jr., M.D.
Medical Director
North Shore Children's Hospital
Salem, Massachusetts
Assistant Professor of Pediatrics
Tufts University School of Medicine
Boston, Massachusetts

Abdollah Sadeghi-Nejad, M.S., M.D., F.A.A.P.
Associate Professor of Pediatrics
Tufts University School of Medicine
Pediatric Endocrinologist
New England Medical Center Hospital
(Boston Floating Hospital for Infants
  and Children)
Boston, Massachusetts

John B. Watkins, M.D.
Director, Division of Gastroenterology
    and Nutrition
Children's Hospital of Philadelphia
Associate Professor of Pediatrics
University of Pennsylvania School of
    Medicine
Philadelphia, Pennsylvania

Shiao Y. Woo, M.D.
Assistant Professor of Pediatrics
Tufts University School of Medicine
Assistant Pediatric
    Hematologist/Oncologist
New England Medical Center Hospital
(Boston Floating Hospital for Infants
    and Children)
Boston, Massachusetts

Introduction

Pediatrics: PreTest Self-Assessment and Review, 3rd Ed. has been designed to provide medical students, as well as physicians, with a comprehensive and convenient instrument for self-assessment and review within the field of pediatrics. The 500 questions provided have been designed to parallel the format and degree of difficulty of the questions contained in Part II of the National Board of Medical Examiners examinations, the Federation Licensing Examination (FLEX), and the Foreign Medical Graduate Examination in the Medical Sciences (FMGEMS).

Each question in the book is accompanied by an answer, a paragraph explanation, and a specific page reference to either a current journal article, a textbook, or both. A bibliography which lists all the sources used in the book follows the last chapter.

Perhaps the most effective way to use this book is to allow yourself one minute to answer each question in a given chapter; as you proceed, indicate your answer beside each question. By following this suggestion, you will be approximating the time limits imposed by the board examinations previously mentioned.

When you have finished answering the questions in a chapter, you should then spend as much time as you need verifying your answers and carefully reading the explanations. Although you should pay special attention to the explanations for the questions you answered incorrectly, you should read every explanation. The authors of this book have designed the explanations to reinforce and supplement the information tested by the questions. If, after reading the explanations for a given chapter, you feel you need still more information about the material covered, you should consult and study the references indicated.

This book meets the criteria for up to 22 credit hours in Category 5(D) for the Physician's Recognition Award of the American Medical Association. It should provide an experience that is instructive as well as evaluative; we also hope that you enjoy it. We would be happy to receive your comments.

General Pediatrics

William F. Rowley, Jr.

DIRECTIONS: Each question below contains five suggested answers. Choose the **one best** response to each question.

1.   After head injuries, the second most common site of trauma causing death in children who are victims of abuse are intraabdominal injuries. These children typically present with all of the following EXCEPT

(A) vomiting
(B) abdominal distension
(C) abdominal tenderness
(D) shock
(E) ecchymoses overlying the abdomen

2.   Accurate estimation of the surface area of a burn requires knowledge of how the body's total surface area is apportioned among the various parts. The chief difference between infants and adults relative to surface area is that infants have a proportionally

(A) smaller surface area for the trunk
(B) smaller surface area for the genitals
(C) smaller surface area for the hands and feet
(D) larger surface area for the head and neck
(E) larger surface area for the buttocks

3.   Of the types of lice that are obligate parasites of humans, the vector of typus, trench fever, and relapsing fever is

(A) *Pediculus humanis capitis*
(B) *Pediculus humanis pedis*
(C) *Pediculus humanis corporis*
(D) *Phthirus pubis*
(E) *Dermacentor andersoni*

4.   Developing a tan is often a preoccupation with adolescents, but there are fungal infections that may interfere with tanning. One is called tinea versicolor and is caused by

(A) *Microsporum audoreini*
(B) *trichophyton mentagnophytes*
(C) *Microsporum tonsurans*
(D) *Pityrosporon orbiculare*
(E) *Trichophyton schoenleni*

5. Although the exact cause of sudden infant death syndrome is unknown, all of the following statements concerning this syndrome are true EXCEPT that

(A) it affects female and male infants equally
(B) it typically involves infants two to four months of age
(C) it is more common among siblings of affected infants
(D) it has a higher incidence among illegitimate infants
(E) it has a higher incidence among infants of lower socioeconomic status

6. The developmental assessment of children is an integral part of pediatric care. At which of the following age intervals should a child be able to run and turn without losing balance, lace shoes (without tying them), and count to 4?

(A) One to two years of age
(B) Two to three years of age
(C) Three to four years of age
(D) Four to five years of age
(E) Five to six years of age

7. Salicylate poisoning, the most common type of accidental poisoning in preschool children, is most likely to be associated with which of the following conditions?

(A) Respiratory acidosis followed by metabolic alkalosis
(B) Respiratory alkalosis followed by metabolic alkalosis
(C) Respiratory alkalosis followed by metabolic acidosis
(D) Metabolic acidosis superimposed upon respiratory alkalosis
(E) Metabolic acidosis superimposed upon respiratory acidosis

8. All of the following are manifestations of chronic hypervitaminosis A EXCEPT for

(A) hepatomegaly
(B) alopecia
(C) desquamation of palms and soles
(D) tender swelling of bones
(E) subcutaneous calcifications

9. To induce vomiting at home in a child who has ingested a poison, the recommended agent of choice would be

(A) copper sulfate
(B) mustard in warm water
(C) apomorphine
(D) fluid extract of ipecac
(E) syrup of ipecac

10. Iridocyclitis (anterior uveitis), which is depicted in the photograph below, is most likely to be associated with which of the following disorders?

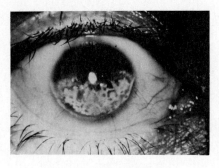

(A) Juvenile rheumatoid arthritis
(B) Slipped femoral epiphysis
(C) Schönlein-Henoch purpura
(D) Legg-Calvé-Perthes disease
(E) Osgood-Schlatter disease

11. Lyme arthritis is usually preceded by a characteristic rash that is

(A) erythema marginatum
(B) urticaria
(C) erythema chronicum migrans
(D) erythema multiforme
(E) morbilliform

12. A buccal smear is performed on a child to determine the presence and number of Barr bodies; the nucleus of a buccal cell is shown below. The sex-chromosome pattern of this child is

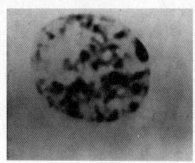

(A) XO
(B) XY
(C) XX
(D) XXX
(E) XXXX

13. The child shown below has been brought to the emergency room because of an inability to urinate. The most likely diagnosis is

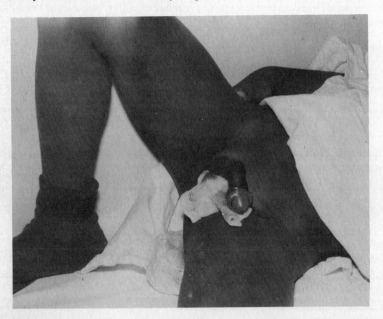

(A) priapism
(B) balanitis
(C) balanoposthitis
(D) phimosis
(E) paraphimosis

14. In children, the most commonly recognized form of familial hyperlipidemia is

(A) hypertriglyceridemia
(B) hypercholesterolemia
(C) hyperchylomicronemia
(D) combined hyperlipidemia
(E) type V hyperlipoproteinemia

15. Osgood-Schlatter disease, one of several disorders classified as osteochondrosis, involves the

(A) tarsal navicular
(B) metatarsal head
(C) capital femoral epiphysis
(D) tibial tuberosity
(E) body of the sternum

16. A six-year-old asthmatic child is brought to the emergency room because of severe coughing and wheezing during the prior 24 hours. The child had been taking ephedrine and theophylline as prescribed without relief and had vomited four times in the last hour. Physical examination reveals a child who is anxious, has intercostal and suprasternal retractions, expiratory wheezing throughout all lung fields, and a respiratory rate of 60 per minute. Initial treatment should include the administration of

(A) intravenous aminophylline
(B) parenteral phenobarbital
(C) subcutaneous epinephrine (Adrenaline)
(D) subcutaneous crystalline epinephrine suspension (Sus-Phrine)
(E) isoproterenol by intermittent positive-pressure breathing

17. Pityriasis rosea is a common, benign cause of rash in children, characterized by a herald patch that usually precedes the generalized eruption. The etiologic agent of the disease is

(A) viral
(B) mycobacterial
(C) fungal
(D) spirochyte
(E) unknown

18. Evaluation of cerebrospinal fluid is critical in evaluating children of all ages for possible central nervous system infections. Normally, the CSF should contain no more than five leukocytes and the protein should be between 10–30 mg/dl. However, in newborns the values are different. Which of the following combinations is most typical?

(A) Up to fifteen leukocytes and 300 mg/dl protein
(B) Up to five leukocytes and less than 10 mg/dl protein
(C) Up to fifteen leukocytes and 100 mg/dl protein
(D) Zero cells and 100 mg/dl protein
(E) Up to 100 red blood cells and 300 mg/dl protein

19. Treatment of child who has acute lead encephalopathy should include prompt administration of

(A) edetate calcium disodium (Ca EDTA)
(B) edetate calcium disodium and dimercaprol (British anti-lewisite)
(C) D-penicillamine
(D) D-penicillamine and dimercaprol
(E) D-penicillamine, edetate calcium disodium, and dimercaprol

Questions 20–21

An eight-month-old girl is admitted to a hospital because of poor weight gain despite a voracious appetite. The presence of steatorrhea and a right upper lobe pneumonia points to cystic fibrosis.

20. If cystic fibrosis is the correct diagnosis, results of her sweat test would be expected to show

(A) low sodium and chloride concentrations
(B) low sodium concentration and high chloride concentration
(C) normal sodium and chloride concentrations
(D) high sodium concentration and normal chloride concentration
(E) high sodium and chloride concentrations

21. The parents of the girl described above want to know whether future offspring also will be born with cystic fibrosis. They should be advised that the chance that their next child will have the disease is approximately

(A) 0 percent
(B) 25 percent
(C) 33 percent
(D) 50 percent
(E) 100 percent

22. The child pictured below has the most common type of generalized skeletal dysplasia. This disorder is

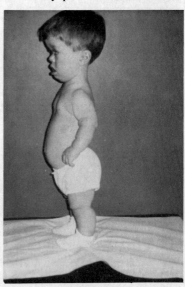

(A) achondrogenesis
(B) achondroplasia
(C) metatropic dwarfism
(D) thanatophoric dwarfism
(E) chondroectodermal dysplasia

23. The bone most frequently fractured at the time of delivery is the

(A) cranium
(B) radius
(C) femur
(D) tibia
(E) clavicle

24. Idiopathic scoliosis most frequently affects

(A) newborn infants
(B) preschool girls
(C) preschool boys
(D) adolescent girls
(E) adolescent boys

DIRECTIONS: Each question below contains four suggested answers of which **one or more** is correct. Choose the answer:

A	if	**1, 2, and 3**	are correct
B	if	**1 and 3**	are correct
C	if	**2 and 4**	are correct
D	if	**4**	is correct
E	if	**1, 2, 3, and 4**	are correct

25. Otitis media occurring during the first six weeks of life deserves special consideration because the bacteria responsible during this time may be different than in older infants and children. Among these organisms are

(1) *Klebsiella pneumoniae*
(2) *Escherichia coli*
(3) *Pseudomonas aeruginosa*
(4) *Hemophilus influenzae*

26. In addition to characteristic skin lesions, Schönlein-Henoch purpura (anaphylactoid purpura) also is associated with which of the following conditions?

(1) Arthritis
(2) Abdominal pain
(3) Nephritis
(4) Paresis

27. Excessive weight gain in a pregnant woman can indicate the presence of which of the following congenital disorders in the fetus?

(1) Anencephaly
(2) Trisomy 18
(3) Duodenal atresia
(4) Renal agenesis

28. Among those entities that cause enlarged testes after puberty is the "fragile X syndrome." Affected males also present with

(1) precocious puberty
(2) penile enlargement
(3) hormonal changes
(4) mental retardation

29. Plumbism (lead intoxication) can be associated with which of the following hematologic findings?

(1) Decreased activity of delta-aminolevulinic acid dehydratase
(2) Decreased level of erythrocyte protoporphyrin
(3) Increased urinary excretion of protoporphyrin
(4) Increased uptake and utilization of iron

30. At 28 weeks of age a normal baby should be able to

(1) sit with support
(2) roll over
(3) utter repetitive vowel sounds
(4) reach for and grasp large objects

SUMMARY OF DIRECTIONS

A	B	C	D	E
1,2,3 only	**1,3** only	**2,4** only	**4** only	**All are correct**

31. Familial dysautonomia (Riley-Day syndrome) is a genetic disease with disturbances in autonomic and sensory functions. This entity is important in the differential diagnosis of a number of chronic problems of childhood, such as

(1) failure to thrive
(2) chronic pulmonary infection
(3) indifference to pain
(4) hypotension

32. Children with cleft palate need to have a team approach if complications are to be avoided. Among the complications that are frequently encountered are

(1) speech disorders
(2) dental caries
(3) malocclusion
(4) otitis media

33. The child pictured below has Down's syndrome. Her surgical scar and purpuric lesions are likely to be associated with

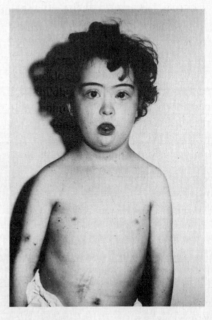

(1) leukemia
(2) thrombotic thrombocytopenic purpura
(3) congenital duodenal atresia
(4) intussusception

34. *Enterobius vermicularis* is a ubiquitous organism that frequently causes more concerns than its medical importance would justify. Among the signs and symptoms that may be related to this parasite's presence are

(1) eosinophilia
(2) anal pruritis
(3) bowel obstruction
(4) sleeplessness

35. Down's syndrome can be associated with which of the following chromosomal patterns?

(1) t(15q21q) centric fusion
(2) 46,XX
(3) Trisomy 21
(4) D/G translocation

36. The infant born to a heroin-addicted mother may show signs of withdrawal as late as four to six weeks after delivery. The signs of withdrawal may include

(1) flapping tremors
(2) diarrhea
(3) flushing
(4) flaccid extremities

37. The increasing use of organophosphate insecticides has led to a rise in the number of organophosphate poisonings. Physical findings associated with organophosphate intoxication can include

(1) tachycardia
(2) muscle fasciculations
(3) hypotension
(4) wheezing

38. Among conditions that cause edema of the eyelids is orbital cellulitis, which is a serious infection that must be recognized early and treated aggressively if complications are to be avoided. The condition is usually associated with which of the following?

(1) Chemosis
(2) Lack of systemic signs
(3) Limitation of movement of the eye
(4) Absence of pain

39. Parents of an eight-month-old infant are concerned about their child's strabismus. They can be informed that

(1) it is most likely due to a refractive error
(2) early identification and treatment improve the outcome
(3) children generally outgrow strabismus
(4) a small degree of strabismus may lead to amblyopia ex anopsia

40. The vitamins that must be provided in the diet to maintain good health include

(1) thiamine
(2) nicotinic acid
(3) folic acid
(4) biotin

41. Teenage pregnancies and their complications are an increasing problem that calls for a comprehensive approach. In teenage pregnancy there is an increased incidence of

(1) preeclampsia and eclampsia
(2) premature delivery
(3) mental retardation in offspring
(4) nutritional disorders

42. Children who have been abused in their home can develop which of the following psychological reactions?

(1) Inability to sustain loving relationships
(2) Tendency to resort to provocation when dealing with loss
(3) Decreased threshold for impulsive behavior
(4) Tendency to seek affectionate attention from sexual contacts

SUMMARY OF DIRECTIONS

A	B	C	D	E
1,2,3 only	1,3 only	2,4 only	4 only	All are correct

43. Whereas in older children the pattern of scabies is similar to that seen in adults, the findings in infants differ in which of the following ways?

(1) Bullae and pustules are common
(2) Burrows are absent
(3) Palms and soles are often involved
(4) Face is spared

44. Anorexia nervosa, which is increasing in frequency, is associated with which of the following symptoms?

(1) Decreased pulse rate
(2) Hyperactivity
(3) Diminished leukocyte count
(4) Increased body temperature

45. Which of the following clinical signs can help differentiate acute otitis externa from acute otitis media?

(1) Pain heightened by movement of the tragus
(2) A red tympanic membrane
(3) Preauricular adenitis
(4) A foul-smelling discharge

46. Type I homocystinuria and Marfan's syndrome have many similar clinical findings, and their ultimate differentiation is sometimes based upon laboratory data. Which of the following features is NOT associated with both syndromes?

(1) Abnormal skeletal appearance
(2) Cardiovascular problems
(3) Ectopia lentis
(4) Mental retardation

DIRECTIONS: The groups of questions below consist of lettered choices followed by several numbered items. For each numbered item select the **one** lettered choice with which it is **most** closely associated. Each lettered choice may be used once, more than once, or not at all.

Questions 47–51

For each disorder that follows, select the dietary deficiency that is most likely to be responsible.

(A) Caloric deficiency
(B) Thiamine deficiency
(C) Niacin deficiency
(D) Vitamin D deficiency
(E) None of the above

47. Marasmus

48. Kwashiorkor

49. Pellagra

50. Beriberi

51. Rickets

Questions 52–55

For each of the following syndromes that can cause childhood deafness, select the clinical finding with which it is most likely to be associated.

(A) Pulmonary stenosis
(B) White forelock
(C) Goiter
(D) Retinitis pigmentosa
(E) Polydactyly

52. Waardenburg's syndrome

53. Pendred's syndrome

54. Usher's syndrome

55. Leopard syndrome

Questions 56–60

Some of the numerous forms of dwarfism recognizable at birth or within the newborn period have distinguishing features that are useful in differential diagnosis. For each distinguishing feature listed below, select the disorder with which it is most likely to be associated.

(A) Achondrogenesis
(B) Diastrophic dwarfism
(C) Thanatophoric dwarfism
(D) Chondrodystrophia calcificans congenita
(E) Chondroectodermal dysplasia

56. Marked micromelia

57. Congenital heart disease

58. Flattened vertebral bodies

59. Natal teeth

60. Swollen ears

Questions 61–66

Drug and alcohol abuse is a problem that endangers a significant percentage of the adolescent population in the United States. For each of the specific drugs listed below that are currently abused, select the class to which it most likely belongs.

(A) Opiates
(B) Hallucinogens
(C) Cannabis
(D) Stimulants
(E) Hypnotic sedatives

61. Marihuana

62. Phencyclidine

63. Alcohol

64. Cocaine

65. Heroin

66. Mescaline

Questions 67–70

For each disorder listed below, select the age and sex distribution with which it is most likely to be associated.

(A) Males 4 to 10 years of age
(B) Males 13 to 18 years of age
(C) Females 4 to 10 years of age
(D) Females 10 to 16 years of age
(E) None of the above

67. Legg-Calvé-Perthes disease

68. Slipped capital femoral epiphysis

69. Idiopathic scoliosis

70. Subluxation of the head of the radius

General Pediatrics
Answers

1.   The answer is E. *(Behrman, ed 12. pp 99–104.)* In addition to the signs A-D listed in the question, a child who has been physically abused, may present with absent bowel sounds. However, the overlying skin is often free of bruises because the abdominal wall is flexible and the force of the blow is transmitted to the internal organs. Rupture of the liver or spleen is the most common finding. Intramural hematomas of the duodenum and proximal jejunum may lead to signs of obstruction, and even chylous ascities and pseudocyst of the pancreas have been reported.

2.   The answer is D. *(Rudolph, ed 17. p 719.)* The percentage of total surface area taken up by the head and neck of a one-year-old child is almost twice that for the same region in a ten-year-old child and nearly three times that in an adult. The percentage of surface area of the hands, feet, trunk, and genitals remains fairly constant despite the overall increase in total surface area. The surface area of the buttocks is proportionally less in an infant than in an adult.

3.   The answer is C. *(Behrman, ed 12. pp 1725–1726.)* Of the three types of lice that are obligate parasites of humans, *Pediculus humanis capitis, Phthirus pubis,* and *Pediculus humanis corporis,* only the body louse, *Pediculus humanis corporis,* is a vector for typhus, trench fever, and relapsing fever. Pediculosis capitis may cause intense pruritus, and secondary infection is common; although the lice may not be seen, the nits may be found attached firmly to hairs, particularly in the occipital region and above the ears. While pediculosis pubis is usually encountered among adolescents, young children may occasionally acquire the disease through close contact. Pediculosis corporis is usually associated with poor hygiene since the lice are most often transmitted via infested clothing or bedding, the nits and lice collecting in the seams of the cloth. Gamma benzene hydrochloride, in lotion or shampoo form, is effective for all three types of lice. Clothing and bedding should be carefully laundered.

4. The answer is D. *(Behrman, ed 12. pp 1715–1716.)* Tinea versicolor is a common chronic fungal infection of the skin caused by *Pityrosporon orbiculare (Malassezia furfur)*, which exists as a part of the normal flora. However, with excessive sweating, debilitating disease or genetic predisposition proliferation of filaments occur and the disease state is produced. The lesions vary widely in appearance from reddish-brown in caucasians to hyper- or hypopigmented in deeply pigmented persons. The lesions begin as macules covered with fine scales and may converge to form patches; they occur mainly on the neck, chest, upper back, and face. There is often little or no pruritus, and the involved areas do not tan following exposure to the sun. Many agents are useful in treatment, such as selenium sulfide preparations and sodium hyposulfite lotions. It should be remembered that this organism is a part of the normal flora, so recurrences are common.

5. The answer is A. *(Kelly, Pediatrics 63:355–360, 1979. Behrman, ed 12. pp 1770–1773.)* The sudden infant death syndrome (crib death, SIDS) typically affects infants two to four months of age and rarely occurs after six months of age. Male infants are affected more frequently than female infants and premature infants more frequently than full-term infants. This syndrome has a higher than normal incidence among infants who are illegitimate or who come from socioeconomically deprived families. Crib deaths tend to recur within families; siblings of affected infants are four to seven times more likely to experience crib death than infants in the general population. However, no distinct genetic pattern has yet been established. The occurrence of periodic breathing (repeated apneic spells) during sleep in infants with near-miss SIDS suggests a causative relationship in some cases.

6. The answer is D. *(Behrman, ed 12. pp 20, 37.)* Children between four and five years of age should be able to run and turn without losing their balance. A three-year-old child may begin to button and unbutton clothing but, unlike a five-year-old child, normally cannot lace up shoes. The concept of numbers shows a similar increase in understanding; children between four and five years of age generally can count to 4, while children one year older are able to count at least to 10.

7. The answer is D. *(Behrman, ed 12. pp 1798–1791.)* The initial symptoms of salicylate poisoning are caused by vagal stimulation of the respiratory center. Minute volume consequently increases, and protraction of the expiratory phase causes the P_{CO_2} to decrease. The respiratory alkalosis thus produced is soon followed by renal compensation, which increases urinary excretion of bicarbonate and decreases loss of chloride, which then cause plasma chloride levels to rise and serum base levels to fall. In addition to these effects, salicylates also interfere with carbohydrate metabolism, and a persistent ketosis develops. Because the ketoacidosis further induces depletion of base through renal excretion, a true metabolic acidosis becomes superimposed upon the respiratory alkalosis. The ingested salicylates account directly for only a small portion of the acidosis; it is their interference with the Krebs cycle that causes accumulation of lactic acid, a more significant factor in the resultant metabolic acidosis. The effect on the Krebs cycle is due to an uncoupling of oxidative phosphorylation. This is also the cause of hyperpyrexia, another manifestation of salicylism, to which unknowing parents often respond with additional salicylates.

8.   The answer is E. *(Behrman, ed 12. p 172.)* Chronic hypervitaminosis A develops due to excessive intake of vitamin A over a period of a month or more. Initial symptoms are nonspecific and include anorexia, pruritus, failure to gain weight, irritability, and tender swelling of bones associated with cortical hyperostosis. Among other manifestations of chronic hypervitaminosis A are hepatomegaly, alopecia, craniotabes, desquamation of palms and soles, seborrheic cutaneous lesions, and signs of increased intracranial pressure, including papilledema and bulging of the fontanelles. Daily intake of vitamin A should be at least 1500 IU for infants and 2000 to 5000 IU for older children.

9.   The answer is E. *(Rudolph, ed 17. p 726.)* Except where emesis is contraindicated, such as in the ingestion of kerosene, syrup of ipecac is the usual treatment of choice in the management of children who have ingested poisons. It is highly effective and, in an oral dose of 15 to 30 ml, usually induces vomiting within 10 to 30 minutes. (It is important not to confuse syrup of ipecac with fluid extract of ipecac, which is highly toxic and should not be kept in the home.) Apomorphine, which must be given by injection, is generally not available in the home, and copper sulfate and tartar emetics are not recommended because of their toxicity. Mustard and warm water is an ineffective emetic preparation. In contrast to induction of emesis, gastric lavage is less effective in removing ingested tablets; moreover, it carries a risk of perforation. Gastric lavage is necessary, however, for treatment of comatose patients. Other important methods for removing ingested poisons include the administration of a cathartic and an adsorbant, activated charcoal.

10. The answer is A. *(Rudolph, ed 17. p 432.)* Up to 25 percent of children who have the monoarticular or pauciarticular form of juvenile rheumatoid arthritis have iridocyclitis as their only significant systemic manifestation. Because this eye disorder may develop without signs or symptoms, it is recommended that all children with this form of arthritis have a slit-lamp eye examination every three months. Iridocyclitis cannot be discovered by regular opthalmoscopic examination.

11. The answer is C. *(Behrman, ed 12. p 586.)* Lyme disease, named for Lyme, Connecticut, is caused by at least two bacterial agents transmitted by tick bite. It usually presents with the rash of erythema chronicum migrans. The rash begins as a small endurated macule or papule on the back, thigh or buttocks, or occasionally in the axilla. The lesion gradually expands to form a large ring with central clearing; subsequently, other similar lesions may occur. The lesions are usually warm and occasionally produce a painful burning sensation. The rash usually lasts about three weeks but may last from just a few days to eight weeks.

Attacks of arthritis, particularly involving the knees and other large joints, may last for months and often recur. Fever, aseptic meningitis, myocardial conduction defects, and cranial nerve palsies may also occur. Treatment is with penicillin or tetracycline.

12. The answer is C. *(Rudolph, ed 17. pp 1542–1543.)* In human somatic cells, only one X chromosome is physiologically active in replication. All additional X chromosomes become inactivated and condensed; these are visible within the nuclei of interphase cells as sex-chromatin bodies (Barr bodies). Thus, the number of sex-chromatin bodies in a cell is one less than the total number of X chromosomes (the Lyon hypothesis). Microscopic examination of a buccal smear from a normal female (XX) would show one Barr body in every cell nucleus, as shown below:

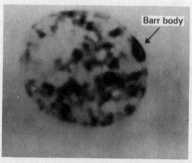

A similar preparation for a normal male (XY) shows no Barr bodies.

13. The answer is E. *(Rudolph, ed 17. p 1216.)* Paraphimosis occurs when a retracted prepuce remains behind the glans; edema develops, preventing reduction of the paraphimosis. If untreated, the disorder can lead to gangrene of the glans. Reduction of the paraphimosis usually necessitates sedation; occasionally, slitting of the constricted ring may be required. All affected children should be circumcised once the inflammation has disappeared. Phimosis is characterized by an inability to retract the foreskin of the penis due to a narrowing of the preputial opening. Balanitis and balanoposthitis are inflammatory disorders affecting the glans penis and, in the case of balanoposthitis, the prepuce; these disorders develop when persistent adhesions between the foreskin and glans penis cause retention of smegma mixed with urine and lead to infection or chemical irritation.

14. The answer is B. *(Rudolph, ed 17. pp 327–328.)* Familial hypercholesterole-mia (classic type II hyperlipoproteinemia) is the most common form of familial hyperlipidemia occurring in childhood. The incidence of affected heterozygotes has been estimated at between 0.2 and 0.5 percent. The disorder is characterized by elevation of total cholesterol as well as low-density lipoprotein cholesterol levels in the plasma. Manifestations of familial hypercholesterolemia include the presence of tendon xanthomas, an increased likelihood of premature ischemic heart disease, and development during childhood of corneal arcus. Although a heterozygous child may be asymptomatic up to the age of ten, homozygous children may have physical signs, particularly planar xanthomas, from birth.

15. The answer is D. *(Behrman, ed 12. p 1622.)* Osgood-Schlatter disease, a juvenile osteochondrosis, is most probably due to repeated trauma to the tibial tuberosity caused by excessive use of the quadriceps muscle. The disease causes pain and swelling over the tibial tubercle and tenderness on palpation. Irregular mineralization of the tibial tubercle is usually visible on x-ray. Avoidance of strenuous activity for one to two months is usually sufficient treatment. If this does not control symptoms, a cast may be required.

16. The answer is C. *(Behrman, ed 12. pp 539–547.)* Children in acute and obvious distress because of an episode of asthma usually respond to treatment with subcutaneous epinephrine (Adrenalin). Two or three injections may be required before symptoms are relieved. Once their asthmatic episodes have abated, affected children may be given a long-acting form of epinephrine, such as crystalline epinephrine suspension (Sus-Phrine), before going home. For children who do not respond to epinephrine, isoproterenol given by intermittent positive-pressure inhalation therapy may prove efficacious. If neither epinephrine nor isoproterenol is effective and respiratory distress persists, the patient should be considered to be in status asthmaticus and hospitalized immediately. Management then includes measurement of arterial blood gases and pH, intravenous administration of aminophylline and corticosteroids, and inhalation therapy with humidified oxygen and bronchodilators. Intravenous hydration and correction of acidosis are essential, and in some children previously unresponsive to epinephrine, may make subsequent injections of epinephrine more effective. Theophylline toxicity should be suspected in children who develop vomiting, irritability, or seizures, and xanthine administration should cease until accurate blood measurements can be obtained. Sedatives, which may cause respiratory depression, are contraindicated in the treatment of children with respiratory distress.

17. The answer is E. *(Behrman, ed 12. pp 1693–1694.)* Pityriasis rosea is a benign eruption of unknown etiology. The lesions may be asymptomatic to severely pruritic. The characteristic "herald patch" usually precedes the general eruption by five to ten days and is a large, solitary, round or oval scaly lesion occurring anywhere on the body. When the generalized eruption occurs, it involves mainly the trunk and proximal limbs. The lesions are usually scaly, less than 1 cm in diameter, oval or round, and pink to brown. The long axis of each lesion is aligned toward cutaneous cleavage lines, which may form a "christmas tree" pattern on the patient's trunk. The eruption usually lasts two to twelve weeks. There is no specific therapy and treatment is symptomatic.

18. The answer is C. *(Behrman, ed 12. p 1555.)* Normally, there should be no red blood cells in the CSE. Their presence may be due to a traumatic lumbar puncture or to a recent subarachnoid hemorrhage. With subarachnoid hemorrhage, the supernatant is xanthochromic and the collecting tubes successfully show equal quantities of RBCs. With traumatic taps there is usually gradual clearing of the RBCs as successive tubes are used and the supernatant is colorless on centrifugation. In the first weeks of life up to 15 leukocytes and 500 RBCs may normally be present and the protein level as high as 100 mg/dl. However, by three months of age the protein level should have fallen below 30 mg/dl.

19. The answer is B. *(Rudolph, ed 17. pp 745–746.)* The three chelating agents used in the United States to treat individuals who have plumbism are edetate calcium disodium (Ca EDTA), dimercaprol (British anti-lewisite), and D-penicillamine. In children having the highest soft-tissue lead content (i.e., those who have acute encephalopathy), chelating agents must be administered in molar amounts in excess of those of the ingested lead; otherwise, the lead may once again disseminate within tissues of the body and cause further toxicity. Both edetate calcium disodium and dimercaprol should be given promptly in the treatment of a child affected with acute lead encephalopathy; D-penicillamine may be administered later during therapy. Careful restriction of parenteral fluids should be maintained so that further increase in cerebral edema does not occur.

20. The answer is E. *(Behrman, ed 12. pp 1089–1090.)* The sweat test remains the most reliable test for cystic fibrosis. In children, chloride levels in sweat that are greater than 60 meq/L are diagnostic of cystic fibrosis; sodium concentrations are approximately 10 meq/L higher. (Results of sweat tests in adults are harder to interpret, because sweat electrolyte concentrations normally are higher in adults than in children.) The mechanism governing this alteration of sweat electrolyte levels in unknown. Glycogen storage disease, vasopressin-resistant diabetes insipidus, untreated adrenal insufficiency, and a type of ectodermal dysplasia are among the small number of disorders that also may be associated with elevation of sweat electrolyte concentrations; none of these conditions, however, is likely to be confused clinically with cystic fibrosis.

21. The answer is B. *(Behrman, ed 12. pp 1086–1099.)* It is believed that cystic fibrosis is inherited as an autosomal recessive trait, and statistical evidence exists to support this contention. As a result, each child born to parents who have had one child with cystic fibrosis has a 25 percent chance of being affected, a 50 percent chance of being a carrier, and a 25 percent chance of not carrying the gene (or genes) at all. Heterozygotes (carriers) for cystic fibrosis are clinically asymptomatic.

22. The answer is B. *(Rudolph, ed 17. pp 359–360.)* Achondroplasia is the most common form of skeletal dysplasia, occurring with an incidence of approximately 1 in every 9000 deliveries. Affected individuals bear a striking resemblance to one another and are identified by their extremely short extremities, prominent foreheads, short, stubby fingers, and a marked lumbar lordosis. Although they go through normal puberty, affected females must have children by cesarean section because of an associated pelvic deformity.

23. The answer is E. *(Behrman, ed 12. pp 360–361.)* The clavicle is the bone most frequently fractured during delivery. This usually occurs when the shoulder is difficult to deliver during vertex presentation or during the delivery of an extended arm in breech presentation. Typically, the infant does not move the arm on the side of the fracture and there may be crepitation irregularity over the fracture site. There may be spasm of the sternocleidomastoid on the side of the fracture, and swelling may obliterate the usually present supraclavicular depression. These fractures often develop a great deal of callus formation within a week. The outcome is very good and treatment is usually simple immobilization of shoulder and arm on involved side.

24. The answer is D. *(Behrman, ed 12. pp 1624–1625.)* Scoliosis, or lateral curvature of the spine, can be divided into two major subgroups. In *functional scoliosis,* the most common type, spinal curvature may result from trauma that produces muscle spasm or, more often, from the presence of a short leg; bending toward the convex aspect of the curve or, for a short leg, placing a lift under the affected leg can correct the disorder. Functional scoliosis does not progress to *structural scoliosis,* the second subgroup. Structural scoliosis, which is a fixed scoliosis that cannot be corrected by bending, may develop due to hemivertebra, paralysis of muscles, fusion of the ribs, neurofibromatosis, infectious or neoplastic disease that destroys vertebrae, or other causes. Most often, however, structural scoliosis is idiopathic, affecting adolescent girls more frequently than other groups. Treatment, which involves mechanical correction and use of appliances such as the Milwaukee brace, has improved significantly the prognosis of children who have idiopathic scoliosis. Screening for idiopathic scoliosis is an important part of the examination of schoolchildren.

25. The answer is E (all). *(Behrman, ed 12. p 409.)* The symptoms of otitis media in the newborn are similar to those of sepsis: nonspecific and sometimes minor, such as poor feeding, lethargy, vomiting, jaundice, irritability, or low fever. The diagnosis is difficult because of the narrow external ear canal and may be based only on decreased mobility of the eardrum. In addition to the pathogens ordinarily associated with acute otitis media in older infants and children (*H. influenzae* and *S. pneumoniae*), *S. aureus,* group B streptococci, *E. coli, K. pneumoniae,* and *P. aeruginosa* are commonly found in infected newborns under six weeks old. Therapy with an appropriate oral antibiotic such as cefaclor may be given if the infant can be observed closely. However, if sepsis is also suspected, parenteral therapy with ampicillin and an aminoglycoside is necessary until culture results become available.

26. The answer is E (all). *(Behrman, ed 12. pp 1338–1340.)* The clinical manifestations of Schönlein-Henoch purpura are due to vasculitis. Acute inflammation in the skin causes characteristic lesions that begin as urticarial wheals or red maculopapules and progress to purpura, usually on the buttocks and legs. An exudate containing lymphocytes, polymorphonuclear leukocytes, eosinophils, and red blood cells tends to accumulate around the small blood vessels of the corium. Inflammation and hemorrhage also may occur at other sites, notably joints, kidneys, the gastrointestinal tract, and the central nervous system. The arthritis associated with Schönlein-Henoch purpura usually involves the larger joints, particularly the knees and ankles. Nephritis can develop and lead to chronic renal disease, and gastrointestinal symptoms, although usually limited to colicky abdominal pain and bleeding, rarely can result in intussusception. Central nervous system involvement is infrequent, but when it does occur corticosteroid therapy is indicated.

27. The answer is A (1, 2, 3). *(Behrman, ed 12. pp 317, 330.)* It is generally presumed that duodenal atresia leads to hydramnios (polyhydramnios) by interference with reabsorption of swallowed amniotic fluid. Abnormal production or release of antidiuretic hormone by fetuses who have anomalies of the central nervous system is considered to be responsible for hydramnios during their gestations. Hydramnios also is associated with approximately 80 percent of infants who have trisomy 18. Oligohydramnios occurs in association with congenital abnormalities of the fetal kidneys, such as renal agenesis, that inhibit formation of fetal urine.

28. The answer is D (4). *(Behrman, ed 12. pp 1500–1501.)* An association between mental retardation and enlargement of testes occurs in the "fragile X syndrome." The testes reach 30 to 40 ml in size after puberty, and many of these patients have a fragile site at the end of the long arm of the X chromosome. The penis is of normal size, and there are no known hormonal changes. In those families with macroorchidism associated with X-linked mental retardation it is important to identify affected boys by chromosomal analysis in order to do genetic counseling.

29. The answer is B (1, 3). *(Rudolph, ed 17. p 741.)* Lead disrupts the production of hemoglobin by inhibiting several steps in the manufacture of heme. In addition to decreased activity of delta-aminolevulinic acid dehydratase and increased excretion of delta-aminolevulinic acid in the urine, lead poisoning leads to increased erythrocyte protoporphyrin levels and decreased uptake and utilization of iron. Lead also interferes with the synthesis of globin in maturing erythrocytes. As a result of these impairments, a hypochromic, microcytic anemia ensues and basophilic stippling of red blood cells occurs. Red blood cell survival time is shortened and a very mild hemolytic anemia may result.

30. The answer is E (all). *(Behrman, ed 12. pp 16–19.)* A 28-week-old infant should be able to sit briefly with pelvic support, roll over, reach for and hold large objects, and utter vowel sounds. At 40 weeks of age, an infant should creep or crawl, sit up without support, and make consonant sounds in a repetitive fashion ("dada," "mama"). At about one year, infants generally are able to walk with assistance. Evaluation of a child's development can be affected by a variety of circumstances, such as hunger, fatigue, or illness, which can impede a child's performance. Serial examinations are therefore much more reliable in assessing accurately a child's development.

31. The answer is A (1, 2, 3). *(Behrman, ed 12. pp 1598–1599.)* The Riley-Day syndrome, inherited as autosomal recessive, is most common in Ashkenazi Jews and has a variety of clinical manifestations. Poor coordination of swallowing movements may lead to repeated episodes of vomiting, gagging, and aspiration. The aspirations may set the stage for repeated pulmonary infections with eventual development of cor pulmonale, or chronic pulmonary failure, which is the most common cause of death. Other manifestations of autonomic system dysfunction include increased sweating, labile hypertension, and poor temperature control. Disturbances in pain sensation lead to repeated trauma, and absence of corneal sensation increases the chances for development of corneal ulceration. The diagnosis is suggested by the finding of a smooth tongue as a result of diminished or absent taste buds. There is also no production of the characteristic flare when the histamine skin test is performed. There is no specific treatment, but the control of respiratory infections and the prevention of aspiration, corneal ulceration (with artificial tears), dehydration, and injuries may prolong the child's life considerably.

32. The answer is E (all). *(Behrman, ed 12. pp 881–882.)* The incidence of isolated cleft palate is approximately 1 in every 2,500 births. The incidence of cleft lip, with or without cleft palate, is approximately 1 in every 1,000 births. Speech defects can result or persist even after adequate surgical closure of the palate cleft. They are due to a failure of the palatal and pharyngeal muscular structures to produce an adequate valve between the nasopharynx and the oropharynx. Therefore, not enough pressure is built up to produce certain sounds, such as "s", "sh" and "ch." This valve mechanism also fails to be brought into play during swallowing thus preventing adequate closure of the Eustachian tube, which makes the development of otitis media and subsequent hearing problems a persistent problem for many of these children. Dental caries are also a major problem for these children and require constant surveillance. A team approach is frequently needed to treat adequately the comprehensive needs of these children and to provide the support and guidance for the patients, their parents, and their pediatricians.

33. The answer is B (1, 3). *(Behrman, ed 12. pp 295–299.)* Down's syndrome is a major cause of clinically identifiable mental retardation. Affected children show moderate to severe retardation and have a variety of morphologic abnormalities. A small, flattened skull, an upward cast to the eyes, the presence of epicanthic folds, and a protruding tongue contribute to their characteristic facies. These children have a high incidence of duodenal atresia, which must be corrected surgically during the newborn period to relieve intestinal obstruction. Children who have Down's syndrome also have a higher incidence of congenital heart disease. First signs of leukemia, which is 10 to 20 times more likely to occur in Down's syndrome children than in the general population, may be petechiae and bruises, which occur because the uncontrolled proliferation of leukocytes in the bone marrow suppresses platelet production.

34. The answer is C (2, 4). *(Behrman, ed 12. p 858.)* *Enterobius vermicularis* (pinworm) infestation occurs in all regions of the world and particularly affects children between the ages of 5 and 14 years. Humans are infected by the ingestion of eggs carried under fingernails or in bedding, house dust or food. The eggs hatch in the stomach and the larvae migrate to the cecal region where they become adult worms. The females migrate at night to the perianal region and deposit their eggs, leading to sleeplessness and itching. Diagnosis is made by discovery of eggs or worms upon microscopic examination of transparent adhesive tape pressed against the perianal area before waking. Although cleanliness is important, there is no proof that it plays a role in the control of the pinworms, and much of the social anxiety needs to be down-played as the infestation is essentially harmless except for a rare case of appendicitis or vaginitis. There is no tissue invasion nor is eosinophilia noted. A single dose of 100 mg mebendazole is recommended therapy, and often the entire family is treated.

35. The answer is E (all). *(Rudolph, ed 17. pp 242–243.)* Children who have Down's syndrome most commonly have trisomy 21; translocations, especially between D-group and G-group chromosomes — t(15q21q) centric fusion is the most common of these abnormalities — account for a small percentage of cases. Children who have trisomy 21, which is caused by nondisjunction, have 47 chromosomes; karyotypes of children with a translocation reveal a normal chromosome count of 46. The chromosomal defect causing translocation Down's syndrome can be carried by asymptomatic individuals, if the translocation is balanced (i.e., if the amount of chromosomal material is normal, regardless of structural changes in the chromosomes). Therefore, chromosome analysis should be performed on members of an affected child's family, because the chance that future siblings will have Down's syndrome is significantly greater if translocation rather than nondisjunction is the etiology.

36. The answer is A (1, 2, 3). *(Behrman, ed 12. pp 394–395.)* The great majority of infants born to mothers addicted to heroin show clinical manifestations within the first 48 hours after birth; some, however, present as late as four to six weeks of age. The infants are very irritable and usually have tremors that may be fine but are often coarse and flapping. Their extremities are hyperreflexic and stiff. They often have a high-pitched cry, diarrhea, myoclonic jerks, and convulsions. The diagnosis is usually a clinical one based on history and symptoms. Treatment using a variety of regimens of narcotics and sedatives has been successful.

37. The answer is C (2, 4). *(Rudolph, ed 17. pp 183–195.)* When the clinical signs of constricted pupils, bradycardia, and muscle fasciculations are associated with the sudden onset of neurological symptoms, progressive respiratory distress, diaphoresis, diarrhea, and overabundant salivation, a diagnosis of organophosphate poisoning should be suspected. Intake of organophosphate agents can occur by ingestion, inhalation, or absorption through skin or mucosa. Organophosphates inhibit carboxylic esterase enzymes, including acetylcholinesterase and pseudocholinesterase; toxicity depends primarily on the inactivation or inhibition of acetylcholinesterase.

Treatment consists of gastric lavage, if the poison has been ingested, or decontamination of the skin, if exposure has been through contact; maintenance of adequate ventilation and fluid and electrolyte balance also is indicated. All symptomatic children should receive atropine and, if severely affected, cholinesterase reactivating oximes as well. Cholinesterase reactivating oximes quickly restore consciousness by inhibiting the muscarinic and nicotiniclike synaptic actions of acetylcholine. Two cholinesterase reactivating oximes are pralidoxime iodide (PAM) and pralidoxime chloride (Protopam).

38. The answer is B (1, 3). *(Behrman, ed 12. pp 1767–1768.)* Orbital cellulitis is a serious infection of the tissues of the orbit and is characterized by edema of the conjunctivae, proptosis, limitation of movement of the eye, erythema and swelling of the eyelids, pain, and systemic signs such as fever. Orbital cellulitis may follow directly from a wound, or bacteremia, but the most common path is by extension from the paranasal sinuses. The organisms most frequently involved as pathogens are *Haemophilus influenzae, Staphylococcus aureus,* group A beta-hemolytic streptococci, and *Streptococcus pneumoniae.* The risk of complications is great, with extension resulting in loss of vision, cavernous sinus thrombosis, meningitis, or brain abscess. Prompt hospitalization and parenteral antibiotic therapy is indicated.

39. The answer is C (2, 4). *(Rudolph, ed 17. pp 1809–1811.)* Up until the age of about four months, transient strabismus in an infant need not be a cause for concern; however, transient strabismus in older infants or persistent strabismus in any individual warrants detailed opthalmologic evaluation. Although the majority of cases of strabismus are due to faulty innervation of the rectus muscles, refractive errors and a number of intraocular diseases such as retinoblastoma and toxocariasis must be excluded. As an affected child becomes older, strabismus may appear to improve due to a decrease in convergence; children do not outgrow strabismus, however, and the risk of failure to develop binocular vision persists, even in cases of slight deviation. In children who have double vision, progressive loss of vision in the weaker eye (amblyopia ex anopsia) can occur. One of the leading causes of blindness, amblyopia ex anopsia is almost always avoidable and may be reversed if strabismus is recognized and treated before six year of age. Treatment consists of forcing children to use their weak eye (e.g., by patching or medicational mydriasis of the stronger eye) and of restoring binocular vision by surgical or optical corrections.

40. The answer is B (1, 3). *(Rudolph, ed 17. pp 735–737.)* Vitamins can be divided into three groups: obligatory vitamins (vitamin A, thiamine, riboflavin, pyridoxine, folic acid, vitamin B_{12}, vitamin C, and vitamin D), which must be provided in the diet in order to maintain good health; conditional vitamins (nicotinic acid, choline, and vitamin K), which are required only if certain other nutrients are deficient; and questionable vitamins (including inositol, biotin, pantothenic acid, and vitamin E), which have not yet been proven to be essential dietary components.

41. The answer is E (all). *(Behrman, ed 12. pp 61–62.)* The main obstetric complications of teenage pregnancy are preeclampsia and eclampsia, which are thought to be due to inadequate prenatal care and nutrition. The rate of prematurity is high, and this in turn is thought to account for the increased incidence of mental retardation among children of teenage mothers. The incidence of repeat pregnancy is high, and too few communities make provisions for the mother to continue her education. A combination of medical, social, psychological, and educational resources must be made available to permit optimum health and development of the teenage mother and her child.

42. The answer is E (all). *(Rudolph, ed 17. pp 766–768.)* Battered children may be more permanently wounded psychologically than physically. Children who have been abused suffer multiple losses and, as a result, are fearful of personal closeness. These children are unable to forge lasting relationships and later look to their sexual contacts for affection. Tendencies toward provocative and impulsive behavior also are common, and abused children may subsequently abuse their own children. It is imperative that physicians recognize that these factors may contribute to additional physical and psychological injuries and that the provoking child may urgently need psychological assessment and therapy.

43. The answer is A (1, 2, 3). *(Behrman, ed 12. pp 1723–1725.)* Scabies, caused by the mite *Sarcoptes scabiei* var. *hominis,* has recently been increasing among all age groups. Most older children and adults present with intensely pruritic wheals, papules, vesicles and threadlike burrows in the interdigital areas, groin, elbows, and ankles; the palms, soles, face, and head are spared. However, infants usually present with bullae and pustules and the areas spared in adults are often involved in infants. Because of the potential neurotoxic effect to infants of gamma benzene hexachloride due to precutaneous absorption, an alternative should be used, such as 10% crotamiton lotion or cream or a 6% sulfur ointment.

44. The answer is A (1, 2, 3). *(Rudolph, ed 17. p 72.)* Anorexia nervosa, a sometimes life-threatening disorder that primarily affects preadolescent and adolescent girls, is characterized by profound weight loss (25 to 30 percent or more of body weight). Despite vigorous investigation, no organic basis for anorectic weight loss has been found. Affected individuals have a distorted body image and are preoccupied with food. Body temperature may be as low as 35.6°C (96°F); pulse rate, blood pressure, and leukocyte count also are decreased. Anorectic individuals are hyperactive and expend a tremendous amount of energy. Therapy is difficult; skillful psychotherapeutic management is fundamental.

45. The answer is B (1, 3). *(Behrman, ed 12. pp 1024–1025.)* The pain of otitis externa but not of otitis media is increased by movement of the tragus. In addition, the presence of preauricular, postauricular, or cervical adenitis, a feature of outer-ear but not middle-ear disease, aids in making the proper diagnosis. The tympanic membrane, if visualized in otitis externa, may appear normal or red; a red tympanic membrane also characterizes acute suppurative otitis media. The presence of a foul-smelling discharge may occur in association with either otitis externa or otitis media, following rupture of a tympanic membrane.

46. The answer is D (4). *(Behrman, ed 12. pp 428–429, 1167.)* About 50 percent of individuals with type I homocystinuria are mentally retarded, but this is not part of the clinical spectrum in patients with Marfan's syndrome. They both tend to develop dislocation of the lens and a peculiar tall body habitus, with especially long, thin, tapering extremities. Cardiovascular problems are common to both. With a homocystinuria, individuals may develop thromboembolic episodes because of abnormalities in intravascular clotting. Those with Marfan's syndrome often have congenital malformations with progressive dilatation beginning at the aortic valve. This results in aortic regurgitation and an eventual dissecting aneurysm with medial cystic necrosis, which is often the cause of death. Patients with homocystinuria can be detected by the presence of homocystine in the urine by the cyanide-nitroprusside test. Type I homocystinuria is due to deficiency of the enzyme cystathionine synthase. Some of the patients with defects in cystathionine synthase respond clinically to large doses of vitamine B_6 and to methionine restriction.

47–51. The answers are: 47-A, 48-E, 49-C, 50-B, 51-D. *(Behrman, ed 12. pp 166–168, 172–175, 1653–1656.)* Marasmus (infantile atrophy) is due to inadequate caloric intake that may be linked with such factors as insufficient food resources, poor feeding techniques, metabolic disorders, and congenital anomalies. Symptoms of marasmus include progressive weight loss, constipation, muscular atrophy, loss of skin turgor, hypothermia, and edema. In advanced disease, affected infants are lethargic and suffer from starvation diarrhea, which is characterized by the presence of small, mucus-containing stools.

Kwashiorkor, which is caused by a severe deficiency of protein, is the most common — and most serious — type of malnutrition in the world. Caloric intake in affected children may be adequate. Children who have protein deficiency become more susceptible to infection; vomiting, diarrhea, muscle wasting, dermatitis, hepatosplenomegaly, edema, dyspigmentation of the skin and hair, and changes in mental status are among the many manifestations of this disease. The most important laboratory finding is a decrease in serum albumin level.

Pellagra, which literally means "rough skin," is due to a deficiency of niacin. Niacin is an essential component of two enzymes — nicotinamide adenine dinucleotide (NAD) and nicotinamide adenine dinucleotide phosphate (NADP) needed for electron transfer and glycolysis. Pellagra is most prevalent in areas that rely on corn as a basic foodstuff (corn contains little tryptophan, which can be converted into niacin). The classic ("3-D") triad of clinical symptoms of pellagra consists of dermatitis, diarrhea, and dementia.

Beriberi results from a deficiency of thiamine, which is essential for the synthesis of acetylcholine and for the operation of certain enzyme systems in carbohydrate metabolism. Thiamine is present in fair amounts in cereals, fruits, vegetables, and eggs; meat and legumes also are good sources. Thiamine is destroyed by heat, and polishing of grains reduces their thiamine content by removing the coverings that contain most of the vitamin. Clinical disturbances stemming from thiamine deficiency are congestive heart failure, peripheral neuritis, and psychic disturbances.

Rickets is a disorder of bone characterized by defective mineralization — despite normal formation — of collagen, matrix, and osteoid. The type of rickets that responds to administration of normal doses of vitamin D is termed vitamin D-deficient rickets; children who have vitamin D-resistant rickets or rickets due to chronic renal disease are not helped by vitamin D therapy. Deficiency of vitamin D can lead to osseous changes, such as enlargement of the costochondral junctions ("rachitic rosary") and crainotabes, within a few months; advanced rickets may cause scoliosis, pelvic and leg deformities, "pigeon breast," rachitic dwarfism, and other disorders.

52–55. The answers are: 52-B, 53-C, 54-D, 55-A. *(Rudolph, ed 17. p 891.)* Waardenburg's syndrome is the most common of several syndromes that are characterized by both deafness and pigmentary changes. Features of this syndrome, which is inherited as an autosomal dominant disorder, include a distinctive white forelock, heterochromia, unilateral or bilateral congenital deafness, and lateral displacement of the inner canthi.

Individuals who have Pendred's syndrome, inherited as an autosomal recessive trait, typically have a marked hearing loss and thyroid dysfunction. Goiter, which usually develops before affected children reach the age of ten years, may arise because their thyroid glands are unable to convert inorganic iodine into organic iodine. The benign goiter responds to thyroid replacement therapy.

Congenital deafness is also a symptom of the autosomal-recessive Usher's syndrome. Pigmentary changes in the retina (retinitis pigmentosa) can be detected in affected infants, and these degenerative changes continue throughout life. Early visual impairments include loss of night vision and development of tunnel vision. Functional blindness can arise in affected adolescents and adults.

Leopard syndrome is characterized by the presence of multiple lentigines, ocular hypertelorism, pulmonary stenosis, abnormal genitalia, retardation of growth, and profound deafness. The syndrome is inherited as an autosomal dominant disorder with variable penetrance.

56–60. The answers are: 56-A, 57-E, 58-C, 59-E, 60-B. *(Behrman, ed 12. pp 1637–1641.)* Achondrogenesis is a lethal chondrodystrophy which is associated with severe micromelia, a relatively large head, and a narrow trunk.

Diastrophic dwarfism, another type of short-limbed dwarfism, is distinguishable by the swelling of the pinna that appears within the first three weeks of life and persists for three to four weeks, leaving the ears with thick, firm, deformed cartilage. The disease is inherited as an autosomal recessive trait and intelligence is normal in affected children.

Chondrodystrophia calcificans congenita (Conradi disease) is frequently associated with cataracts and optic atrophy. These children may also suffer from seborrheic dermatitis or ichthyosiform erythroderma. The radiologic finding of discrete, multiple calcified densities in those bones formed in hyaline cartilage helps to establish the diagnosis.

Children with thanatophoric dwarfism are born with hypotonia and rapidly develop respiratory distress and asphyxia due to severe narrowing of the thorax. Characteristic x-ray findings include marked flattening of the vertebral bodies.

Chondroectodermal dysplasia (Ellis-van Creveld syndrome) has an unusually high incidence among the Amish, although cases among non-Amish people have also been reported. Anomalies occur in these children in all the embryonic layers of development. Ectodermal abnormalities include fine, sparse hair, dystrophic nails, and peg-shaped teeth with abnormal spacing. Natal teeth are frequently present. Mesodermal abnormalities are manifested by bone involvement resulting in dwarfism, congenital heart disease, and renal malformation. Polydactylism is usually present in these children, who have normal intelligence. The disease has an autosomal recessive inheritance. Penetrance is variable and may be manifested by polydactyly as an isolated finding.

61–66. The answers are: 61-C, 62-B, 63-E, 64-D, 65-A, 66-B. *(Behrman, ed 12. pp 1524–1529.)* In 1972, the National Commission on Marihuana and Drug Abuse reported that 7 percent of American youths were regular users of marihuana. Users of this drug may exhibit a variety of behavioral changes from simple euphoria to hallucinations. Users' response time and coordination may be impaired. A 1976 survey revealed that there seemed to be no increase in usage of marihuana in adolescents but that alcohol was assuming greater importance as an addictive substance.

Phencyclidine (PCP, angel dust) is one of the more common hallucinogens available on the "street." Because PCP may cause confusion and a wide variety of hallucinations, it is of especially high risk to individuals prone to psychiatric problems, in whom prolonged psychosis may be produced. Lysergic acid diethylamide

(LSD) and PCP are often the active ingredients in substances sold as mescaline or psilocybin because they are relatively easy to produce.

Alcohol, while regarded by many as simply a beverage, is a depressant which, among other problems, accounts for an increasing number of automobile accidents. It has been reported that as many as 28 percent of adolescents in the United States are problem drinkers.

Cocaine is another stimulant that is increasingly available. Formerly, cocaine was used in combination with heroin, but it is now often used as a primary drug, even though it is very expensive. Dealing in drugs may be the easiest way for an adolescent to meet the cost of drug use.

Heroin, along with methadone and morphine, is an opiate. It is usually injected but occasionally is taken intranasally. Infections at the injection site, hepatitis, endocarditis, and tetanus are among the medical problems encountered in opiate users.

Mescaline, another hallucinogen, is more likely to be LSD or PCP. Prolonged use of hallucinogens may result in disturbed interpersonal relations, poor time and place orientation, and regressive behavior. With abstinence, hallucinogenic flashbacks may recur for months.

67–70. The answers are: 67-A, 68-B, 69-D, 70-E. *(Rudolph, ed 17. pp 1834–1837. Behrman, ed 12. pp 1620–1621, 1624–1625, 1629.)* Legg-Calvé-Perthes disease (coxa plana) is aseptic necrosis and flattening of the capital femoral epiphysis; the cause of this disorder is unknown. Boys between the ages of four and ten years are most frequently affected. Presenting symptoms include a limp, pain in the knee or hip, or limitation of weight bearing.

Slipped capital femoral epiphysis occurs typically in adolescents; the disorder is slightly more common among boys than girls. The etiology is unknown. Onset of this disorder, which is more common in childhood, is gradual; pain referred to the knee is characteristic and may mask the hip pathology. Treatment aims at arresting the slippage by immobilization of the hip through cast or surgical fixation.

Idiopathic scoliosis occurs most frequently in adolescent girls and requires prompt evaluation. Treatment by bracing, spinal fusion, or both is sometimes necessary. Unrecognized prior infection of the nervous system, leading to muscle weakness, may be a factor in some cases of idiopathic scoliosis.

Subluxation of the head of the radius occurs most commonly in children who are two to five years of age and have been jerked forcibly by the hand. Affected children have pain in the elbow and are unable to supinate the forearm. The diagnosis is established if forcible supination of the forearm, while the elbow is stabilized, easily corrects the subluxation.

The Newborn Infant

Joseph L. Kennedy, Jr.

DIRECTIONS: Each question below contains five suggested answers. Choose the **one best** response to each question.

71. In a neonate who has asphyxia, all of the following sequelae could be expected to develop EXCEPT

(A) sustained rise in blood pressure
(B) cardiomegaly and heart failure
(C) cerebral edema and seizures
(D) electrolyte abnormalities
(E) disseminated intravascular coagulation

72. A full-term infant is born after a normal pregnancy; delivery, however, is complicated by marginal placental separation. At 12 hours of age the child, although appearing to be in good health, passes a bloody meconium stool. For determining the etiology of the bleeding, which of the following diagnostic procedures should be performed first?

(A) A barium enema
(B) An Apt test
(C) Gastric lavage with normal saline
(D) An upper gastrointestinal series
(E) A platelet count, prothrombin time, and partial thromboplastin time

73. Which of the following patterns noted on continuous fetal heart rate monitoring warrants immediate delivery of the infant?

(A) Baseline variability with periodic acceleration
(B) Increasing baseline variability (saltatory pattern)
(C) Early deceleration pattern
(D) Late deceleration without baseline variability
(E) Variable deceleration with baseline variability

74. A healthy premature infant who weighs 950 g (2 lb, 1-1/2 oz) is fed undiluted breast milk to provide 120 cal/kg per day. Over ensuing weeks the baby is most apt to develop

(A) hypernatremia
(B) hypocalcemia
(C) blood in the stool
(D) metabolic acidosis
(E) vitamin E deficiency

75. An infant weighing 1400 g (3 lb) is born at 32 weeks gestation in a delivery room that has an ambient temperature of 23.9°C (75°F). Within a few minutes of birth, this infant is likely to exhibit all of the following manifestations EXCEPT

(A) pallor
(B) shivering
(C) a fall in body temperature
(D) increased respiratory rate
(E) metabolic acidosis

76. A primiparous woman whose blood type is O-positive gives birth at term to an infant who has A-positive blood and a hematocrit of 55%. A serum bilirubin level obtained at 36 hours of age is 12 mg/100 ml. Which of the following laboratory findings would be most characteristic of this infant's disease?

(A) An elevated reticulocyte count
(B) A weakly positive direct Coombs' test
(C) Fragmented red blood cells in the blood smear
(D) Nucleated red blood cells in the blood smear
(E) Hematocrit less than 55%

77. Management of infants born to women with hepatitis B (mother HBeAg positive) should include all of the following EXCEPT

(A) hepatitis B immune globulin (HBIG) given intramuscularly soon after birth
(B) hepatitis B vaccine
(C) immediate thorough bathing
(D) isolation
(E) testing infant for hepatitis B surface antigen (HBsAg)

78. A three-day-old infant born at 32 weeks gestation and weighing 1700 g (3 lb, 12 oz) has three episodes of apnea, each lasting 20 to 25 seconds and occurring after a feeding. During these episodes the heart rate drops from 140 to 100 beats per minute and the child remains motionless; between episodes, however, the child displays normal activity. Blood sugar is 50 mg/100 ml and serum calcium is normal. The child's apneic periods most likely are

(A) due to an immature respiratory center
(B) a part of periodic breathing
(C) secondary to hypoglycemia
(D) manifestations of seizures
(E) evidence of underlying pulmonary disease

79. Two infants are born at 36 weeks gestation. Infant A weighs 2600 g (5 lb, 12 oz) and infant B weighs 1600 g (3 lb, 8 oz). Infant B is more likely to have all of the following problems EXCEPT

(A) congenital malformations
(B) low hematocrit
(C) symptomatic hypoglycemia
(D) aspiration pneumonia
(E) future growth retardation

80. Which of the following statements characterizes the late anemia of prematurity?

(A) The platelet count is diminished
(B) The reticulocyte count is elevated
(C) It cannot occur in the presence of a normal serum tocopherol level
(D) It can be prevented by a diet high in polyunsaturated fatty acids
(E) It is often complicated by iron deficiency

81. The infant pictured below is two weeks old. He was delivered at term after a long and difficult labor. He weighted 4200 g (9 lb, 4 oz) at birth. The lesions shown on his arm and back are reddish-purple and indurated. Which of the following diagnoses is most likely to be correct?

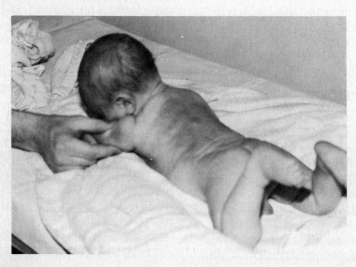

(A) Erythema toxicum neonatorum
(B) Sclerema neonatorum
(C) Subcutaneous fat necrosis
(D) Urticaria pigmentosa
(E) Mongolian spots

82. A one-day-old infant who was born by a difficult forceps delivery is alert and active. However, she does not move her left arm, which she keeps internally rotated by her side with the forearm extended and pronated; she also does not move it during a Moro reflex. The rest of her physical examination is normal. This clinical picture most likely indicates

(A) fracture of the left clavicle
(B) fracture of the left humerus
(C) left-sided Erb-Duchenne paralysis
(D) left-side Klumpke's paralysis
(E) spinal injury with left hemiparesis

83. At 43 weeks gestation a long, thin infant is delivered who is apneic, limp, pale, and covered with "pea soup" amniotic fluid. The first step in the resuscitation of this infant after delivery should be

(A) suction of the trachea under direct vision
(B) artificial ventilation with bag and mask
(C) artificial ventilation with endotracheal tube
(D) administration of 100 percent oxygen by mask
(E) catheterization of the umbilical vein

84. Which of the following statements about periventricular/ subependymal hemorrhage in newborn infants is true?

(A) Clinical manifestations appear within minutes of a serious hypoxic episode
(B) It most commonly produces sudden severe neurologic deterioration
(C) It is seldom found in infants weighing less than 1500 g
(D) Systemic signs include an acute drop in hematocrit and arterial P_{O_2} and a marked fall in pH
(E) Posthemorrhagic ventricular dilatation cannot be evaluated adequately except by CAT scan

85. Initial examination of a full-term infant weighing less than 2500 g (5 lb, 8 oz) shows edema over the dorsum of her hands and feet. Which of the following findings would support a diagnosis of Turner's syndrome?

(A) A liver palpable to 2 cm below the costal margin
(B) Tremulous movements and ankle clonus
(C) Redundant skin folds at the nape of the neck
(D) A transient, longitudinal division of the body into a red half and a pale half
(E) Softness of the parietal bones at the vertex

Questions 86–88

After an uneventful labor and delivery, an infant is born at 32 weeks gestation weighing 1500 g (3 lb, 5 oz). Respiratory difficulty develops immediately after birth and increases in intensity thereafter. The child's mother (gravida 3, para 2, no abortions) previously lost an infant because of hyaline membrane disease.

86. At six hours of age the child's respiratory rate is 60 per minute. Examination reveals grunting, intercostal retraction, nasal flaring, and marked cyanosis in room air. Physiologic abnormalities compatible with these data include

(A) decreased lung compliance, reduced lung volume, left-to-right shunt of blood
(B) decreased lung compliance, reduced lung volume, right-to-left shunt of blood
(C) decreased lung compliance, increased lung volume, left-to-right shunt of blood
(D) normal lung compliance, reduced lung volume, left-to-right shunt of blood
(E) normal lung compliance, increased lung volume, right-to-left shunt of blood

87. At eight hours of age the infant is given 70 percent oxygen. Arterial blood gases are as follows: pH, 7.30; P_{O_2}, 44 mmHg; and P_{CO_2}, 56 mmHg. Which of the following therapeutic courses of action would be most appropriate?

(A) Elevation of the inspired oxygen concentration
(B) Initiation of mechanical ventilation
(C) Elevation of the inspired oxygen concentration and administration of sodium bicarbonate
(D) Initiation of continuous positive airway pressure and administration of sodium bicarbonate
(E) Initiation of mechanical ventilation and administration of sodium bicarbonate

88. At 48 hours of age and after proper therapy has been instituted, the infant described is much improved. With the child breathing 70 percent oxygen (without any ventilatory assistance), arterial blood gases are as follows: pH, 7.36; P_{O_2}, 210 mmHg; P_{CO_2}, 40 mmHg. On evaluating this information, the child's physician should

(A) lower the inspired oxygen concentration to 40 percent and, one hour later, repeat arterial puncture for blood gas values
(B) lower the inspired oxygen concentration to 40 percent and, four hours later, repeat arterial puncture for blood gas values
(C) lower the inspired oxygen concentration gradually keeping the transcutaneous P_{O_2} (TcP_{O_2}) less than 90 mmHg
(D) lower the inspired oxygen concentration to 60 percent and, four hours later, repeat arterial puncture for blood gas values
(E) leave the inspired oxygen concentration at 70 percent and, one hour later, repeat arterial puncture for blood gas values.

89. Very shortly after birth, an infant develops abdominal distension and begins to drool constantly. When she is given her first feeding, formula runs out the side of her mouth and she coughs and chokes. Physical examination a few hours later reveals tachypnea, intercostal retractions, and bilateral pulmonary rales.

The esophageal anomaly that most commonly causes the signs and symptoms exhibited by this infant is illustrated by

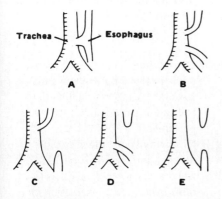

(A) figure A
(B) figure B
(C) figure C
(D) figure D
(E) figure E

90. Failure to administer vitamin K prophylactically to a newborn infant is associated with which of the following?

(A) A deficiency of factor V
(B) A prolonged prothrombin time
(C) Development of hemorrhagic manifestations within 24 hours of delivery
(D) Manifestations that are more severe in male than female infants
(E) A greater likelihood of developing symptoms if the infant is fed cow's milk rather than breast milk

91. A cold, dusky face in a newborn infant can be associated with all of the following EXCEPT

(A) cold stress
(B) hypothyroidism
(C) patent ductus arteriosus
(D) tight nuchal cord
(E) face presentation

92. Which of the following drugs given during the last two weeks of pregnancy is most likely to have deleterious effects on the fetus?

(A) Propanalol
(B) Penicillin
(C) Aluminum hydroxide
(D) Hydantoin
(E) Heparin

93. At the time of delivery of her child, a woman is noted to have a large volume of amniotic fluid. At six hours of age her baby begins regurgitating small amounts of mucus and bile-stained fluid. Physical examination of the infant is normal, and an abdominal x-ray is obtained (shown below). The most likely diagnosis of this infant's disorder is

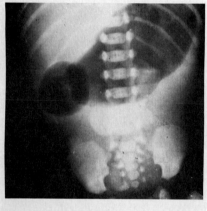

(A) esophageal atresia
(B) pyloric stenosis
(C) gastric duplication
(D) duodenal atresia
(E) midgut volvulus

94. A diagnosis of neonatal necrotizing enterocolitis is confirmed by finding air in the bowel wall (pneumatosis intestinalis) on plain x-ray of an infant's abdomen. Which of the following therapeutic approaches would most likely be recommended?

(A) Immediate surgical resection of affected loops of bowel
(B) Reduction of the volume of feedings and administration of oral and systemic antibiotics
(C) Reduction of the volume of feedings, administration of oral and systemic antibiotics, and careful observation for bowel perforation
(D) Discontinuation of feedings, administration of intravenous fluids and oral and systemic antibiotics, and careful observation for bowel perforation
(E) Discontinuation of feedings, administration of intravenous fluids and oral and systemic corticosteroids, and careful observation for bowel perforation

95. A two-week-old premature infant is found to have several milliliters of formula still present in the stomach two hours after being fed. Also noted are gastric distension and the passage of blood-streaked stools. Which of the following historical factors would best support a tentative diagnosis of necrotizing enterocolitis for this infant?

(A) Passage of a thick tenacious meconium plug at 24 hours of age
(B) Severe hyaline membrane disease with anoxic episodes in the first week of life
(C) Hypocalcemia requiring oral calcium supplementation in the first week of life
(D) A maternal history of severe ulcerative colitis
(E) A history of milk-protein allergy in family members

96. Which of the following statements about the infant pictured below is true?

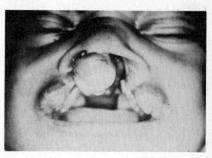

(A) Parenteral alimentation is recommended to prevent aspiration
(B) Surgical closure of the palatal defect should be done before three months of age
(C) Good anatomic closure will preclude the development of speech defects
(D) Recurrent otitis media and hearing loss are likely complications
(E) The chance that a sibling also would be affected is 1 in 1000

97. A woman (gravida 3, para 0, 2 abortions) who is in early labor comes to her community hospital at 34 weeks gestation. The hospital, which has an excellent obstetric service but no intensive-care nursery, is located 25 miles from the nearest referral perinatal center. To maximize the child's chances for survival without causing unnecessary hardship to the woman, which of the following courses of action would be most advisable?

(A) Transfer the woman immediately to the referral perinatal center
(B) Transfer the infant to the referral preinatal center immediately after birth
(C) Transfer the infant to the referral preinatal center at the first sign of illness
(D) Transfer the infant to the referral perinatal center only if a severe illness develops
(E) Keep the woman and her infant at the community hospital

98. The chance of hypoglycemia in the infant of a diabetic mother can be lessened by all of the following EXCEPT

(A) careful control of the maternal blood glucose levels during pregnancy
(B) maternal intravenous loading with 10 percent glucose beginning two to four hours prior to the expected time of delivery
(C) careful glucose monitoring of the infant
(D) intravenous infusion of glucose to the infant in amounts of 6 to 12 mg/kg per minute
(E) maintenance of the infant in a thermo-neutral environment.

99. An infant is born at term to a primigravid woman who has diabetes mellitus. The infant, whose physical examination at birth is normal, is noted at 20 hours of age to be pale and lethargic and to void grossly bloody urine. Physical examination at this time reveals a left flank mass that is firm, lobulated, and about 10 cm in diameter; the mass is opaque on transillumination. The most likely diagnosis is

(A) acute adrenal hemorrhage
(B) retrorenal hematoma
(C) Wilms' tumor
(D) renal vein thrombosis
(E) polycystic kidney

DIRECTIONS: Each question below contains four suggested answers of which **one or more** is correct. Choose the answer:

A	if	**1, 2, and 3**	are correct
B	if	**1 and 3**	are correct
C	if	**2 and 4**	are correct
D	if	**4**	is correct
E	if	**1, 2, 3, and 4**	are correct

100. Physicians using phototherapy to treat an infant who has hyperbilirubinemia secondary to hemolysis should monitor which of the following clinical signs or laboratory values at regular intervals during the 48 hours after initiation of treatment?

(1) Hematocrit
(2) Skin color
(3) Serum bilirubin level
(4) Scleral color

101. Correct statements about hypocalcemia in neonates include which of the following?

(1) It is less likely to occur in breast-fed infants
(2) It is less likely to occur in infants of diabetic mothers
(3) It may be precipitated by obstetric difficulty and asphyxia
(4) It may be partially caused by poor maternal nutrition

102. Correct statements concerning breast-fed infants as compared to bottle-fed infants include which of the following?

(1) Their survival rate in lower socio-economic groups is higher
(2) They tend to be emotionally more stable
(3) They have fewer gastrointestinal disturbances
(4) Their serum bilirubin level during the newborn period is lower

103. In the management of an infant who has hyperbilirubinemia, factors to be considered in assessing the risk of kernicterus include the presence of

(1) acidosis
(2) hypoxia
(3) hypoalbuminemia
(4) cold stress

104. Normal full-term newborn infants can demonstrate which of the following reflex reactions?

(1) Stepping reflex
(2) Palmar grasp
(3) Placing reflex
(4) Parachute reaction

SUMMARY OF DIRECTIONS

A	B	C	D	E
1,2,3 only	1,3 only	2,4 only	4 only	All are correct

105. A 28-year-old primigravid woman, who is unsure of her dates, gives birth to a girl weighing 1900 g (4 lb, 3 oz); this weight is at the 50th percentile for infants born at 33 weeks gestation. Which of the following findings on physical examination would support a gestational age of 33 weeks for this child?

(1) The clitoris is almost hidden by the labia majora
(2) The ear recoils slowly from folding
(3) The elbow can be brought up to the opposite shoulder
(4) The sole has one or two creases over the anterior third

106. An infant born to a heroin addict who has received no prenatal care is likely to exhibit

(1) prematurity and low birth weight
(2) onset of symptoms within the first two days of life
(3) hyperirritability and coarse tremors
(4) vomiting and diarrhea

107. Recent studies on close mother-infant contact in the early postpartum period have yielded findings which include

(1) disturbance by even mild illness of the long-term relationship between mother and infant
(2) evidence that infants hear and respond to their mothers
(3) higher incidence of child abuse and failure-to-thrive in infants not receiving close early contact with their mothers
(4) prolonged breast-feeding in the early-contact group

108. A four-day-old infant has a plasma phenylalanine level greater than 20 mg/100 ml (normal: 0.4 to 2.0); tyrosine levels are normal. Correct statements about this infant include which of the following?

(1) Dietary therapy is needed to prevent mental retardation
(2) Physical examination would be expected to be normal
(3) Both parents are heterozygous
(4) Urine would be positive for phenylpyruvic acid

109. Examination shows that a neonate has a large bulge on the left side of the head; the bulge is sharply demarcated by the coronal, sagittal, and lambdoid sutures. Correct statements concerning this situation include which of the following?

(1) There is a small chance of an underlying skull fracture
(2) Needle aspiration of the swelling is indicated
(3) The lesion is rarely present on the first day of life
(4) If the infant is untreated, a prominent lump will probably persist for many months

110. Correct statements concerning retinopathy of prematurity in newborns include which of the following?

(1) Retinopathy of prematurity is seldom a problem in babies born after 34 weeks gestation
(2) If inspired oxygen concentrations are carefully monitored and controlled, retinopathy of prematurity will not occur
(3) Mild degrees of the condition are manifested as myopia
(4) Vitamin E may prevent the development of proliferative phase.

111. Bronchopulmonary dysplasia is associated with all of the following etiologies EXCEPT

(1) high concentration of oxygen
(2) extreme prematurity
(3) assisted ventilation
(4) meconium aspiration

112. Correct statements describing hypoglycemia affecting infants of diabetic mothers include which of the following?

(1) It is less frequently symptomatic in these infants than in small-for-dates infants
(2) It usually develops in the second day of life
(3) It is believed to be caused by hyperinsulinism
(4) It is best prevented by rapid infusion of a 15 percent glucose solution

113. The diagnosis of meconium ileus in a neonate who has signs of intestinal obstruction is supported by

(1) a family history of cystic fibrosis
(2) palpation of several doughy masses throughout the abdomen
(3) the radiographic presence of unevenly dialated, granular-looking loops of bowel
(4) a greenish discoloration of the abdominal wall

114. A previously healthy full-term infant has several episodes of duskiness and apnea during the third day of life. Diagnostic considerations should include

(1) bacterial meningitis
(2) congenital heart disease
(3) seizure disorder
(4) hypoglycemia

115.   A woman gives birth to twins at 38 weeks gestation. The first twin weighs 2800 g (6 lb, 3 oz) and has a hematocrit of 70%; the second twin weighs 2100 g (4 lb, 10 oz) and has a hematocrit of 40%. Correct statements concerning these infants include which of the following.

(1)   The first twin is at risk for developing respiratory distress, cyanosis, and congestive heart failure
(2)   The first twin may have hyperbilirubinemia and convulsions
(3)   The second twin may be pale, tachycardic, and hypotensive
(4)   The second twin probably had hydramnios of the amniotic sac

116.   A woman pregnant with twins wonders if such pregnancies are associated with an increased risk of infant morbidity or mortality. She should be told that

(1)   second-born twins have a higher mortality rate than first-born twins
(2)   twins are more likely to be born prematurely or to be small for dates
(3)   dichorionic twins have a higher perinatal mortality rate than monochorionic twins
(4)   twins have a fourfold increase in perinatal mortality as compared to singletons

117.   A boy is born at term after an uncomplicated pregnancy, labor, and delivery. Immediately after birth, however, he is noted to be in severe distress, making gasping respiratory efforts accompanied by intercostal retractions. His abdomen is concave, and he is cyanotic. A chest x-ray obtained at this time is shown below. Treatment of this child, whose condition is deteriorating rapidly must include

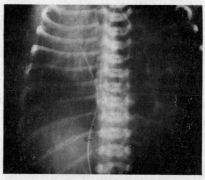

(1)   emergency surgical correction
(2)   prompt correction of metabolic acidosis
(3)   intermittent nasogastric suction
(4)   vigorous positive pressure ventilation

DIRECTIONS: The groups of questions below consist of lettered choices followed by several numbered items. For each numbered items select the **one** lettered choice with which it is **most** closely associated. Each lettered choice may be used once, more than once, or not at all.

Questions 118–121

For each description of congenital anomalies that follows, select the major abnormality with which it is most likely to be associated.

(A) Deafness
(B) Seizures
(C) Wilms' tumor
(D) Congestive heart failure
(E) Optic glioma

118. Nonfamilial bilaterial absence of the iris (aniridia)

119. Heterochromia of the iris, broad nasal root, fusion of the eyebrows, and white forelock

120. Flat capillary hemangioma over the anterior scalp and one side of the face

121. Hypopigmented oval mascules on the skin of the trunk and extremities

Questions 122–125

For each infant described below, select the lettered curve on the graph that best represents the expected course of that infant's jaundice.

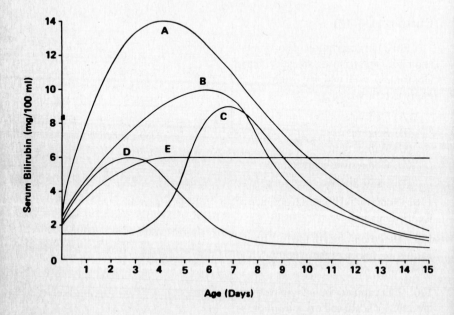

122. A jaundiced premature neonate who is otherwise normal

123. A jaundiced full-term neonate who has septicemia

124. A jaundiced full-term neonate who has hypothyroidism

125. A jaundiced full-term neonate who has erythroblastosis fetalis

The Newborn Infant

Answers

71. The answer is A. *(Avery, ed 2. pp 183–188. Fanaroff, ed 3. pp 191–192.)* During a period of asphyxia, hypoxemia and acidosis and poor perfusion can damage a neonate's brain, heart, kidney, liver, and lungs. The resulting clinical abnormalities include cerebral edema, irritability, seizures, cardiomegaly, heart failure, oligouria or renal failure, poor liver function, and respiratory distress syndrome. Poor perfusion of the lungs may lead to excessively high pulmonary arterial pressure, resulting in a persistent right-to-left shunt across a patent ductus arteriosis or foramen ovale (persistent fetal circulation).

72. The answer is B. *(Avery and Taeusch, ed 5. pp 316–317.)* Hematemesis and melena are not uncommon in the neonatal period, especially if gross placental bleeding has occurred at the time of delivery. The diagnostic procedure that should be done first is the Apt test, which differentiates fetal from adult hemoglobin in a bloody specimen. If the blood in an affected infant's gastric contents or stool is maternal in origin, further workup of the infant is obviated.

73. The answer is D. *(Fanaroff, ed 3. pp 95–107.)* Baseline variability with or without periodic acceleration of the fetal heart rate is a sign of fetal well-being. Increasing baseline variability (saltatory pattern) may represent early compromise of fetal oxygenation. The early deceleration pattern is due to pressure of the anterior fontanel on the cervix and is not a sign of fetal distress. The variable deceleration pattern indicates umbilical cord compression. The late deceleration pattern signifies fetal hypoxemia. Both of these patterns in association with loss of baseline variability are signs of severe fetal compromise and warrant immediate delivery of the infant.

74. The answer is B. *(Fanaroff, ed 3. pp 302–307.)* The average healthy low-birth-weight infant of this size requires a daily intake of 100 to 150 mg/kg of calcium. It is usually impossible with any combination of parenteral and enteral nutrition to match what the infant would have accumulated in utero. Breast milk has less calcium (and phosphorus) than commercial formulas. One may supplement the breast milk with calcium or mix it with commercial formulas designed for the premature infant.

75. The answer is B. *(Avery, ed 2. pp 171–181.)* A room temperature of 24°C (approximately 75°F) provides a cool environment for preterm infants weighing less than 1500 g (3 lb, 4 oz). Aside from the fact that these infants emerge from a warm 37.6° (99.5°F) intrauterine environment, at birth they are wet, have a relatively large surface area for their weight, and have little subcutaneous fat. Within minutes of delivery the infants are likely to become pale or blue and their body temperatures will drop. In order to bring body temperature back to normal they must increase their metabolic rate; ventilation, in turn, must increase proportionally to ensure an adequate oxygen supply. Because a preterm infant is likely to have respiratory problems and be unable to oxygenate adequately, lactate can accumulate and lead to a metabolic acidosis. Infants rarely shiver in response to a need to increase heat production.

76. The answer is E. *(Behrman, ed 12. p 388.)* If a mother has O-positive blood and her baby is A-positive blood, the baby has a 10 percent chance of developing hemolytic disease. Infants who have hemolytic disease due to a major blood-group incompatibility usually are only mildly affected; hyperbilirubinemia is the most frequent complication. Although the hematocrit of affected infants usually is normal, elevation of the reticulocyte count and the presence of nucleated red blood cells and spherocytes in the blood smear provide evidence of hemolysis. In contrast to hemolytic disease due to Rh incompatibility, major blood-group incompatibility is associated with a direct Coombs' test that is most frequently weakly positive.

77. The answer is D(4). *(Lancet 1:939–941, 1984.)* Hepatitis B is the commonest cause of liver disease throughout the world. Vertical transmission from mother to newborn infant is believed to account for up to 40 percent of the world's chronic carriers. The virus does not normally cross the placenta. Infants are usually born HBeAG negative. The infant at risk should be washed thoroughly, given hepatitis B immune globulin (HBIG), and begun on a hepatitis B vaccine schedule with injections at birth, one month and six months. Once this has been accomplished, there is no point in isolation.

78. The answer is A. *(Fanaroff, ed 3. pp 456–460.)* Apneic spells are characterized by an absence of respirations for more than 20 seconds or by bradycardia and cyanosis (or by both). Periods of apnea are thought to be secondary to an incompletely developed respiratory center and are associated most commonly with prematurity. Although seizures, hypoglycemia, and pulmonary disease accompanied by hypoxia all can lead to apnea, these etiologies are unlikely in the infant described, given that no unusual movements occur during the apneic spells, that the blood sugar level is more than 40 mg/100 ml, and that the child appears well between spells. Periodic breathing, a common pattern of respiration in low-birth-weight babies, is characterized by periods of rapid respiration, lasting 10 to 15 seconds, that alternate with periods of apnea, lasting 5 to 10 seconds.

79. The answer is B. *(Fanaroff, ed 3. pp 70–78.)* Small-for-dates infants are subject to a different set of complications than preterm infants whose size is appropriate for gestational age. The small-for-dates infants have a higher incidence of major congenital anomalies and are at increased risk for future growth retardation, especially if length and head circumference as well as weight are small for gestational age. They also are at a greater risk for neonatal asphyxia and the meconium aspiration syndrome, which can lead to pneumothorax, pneumomediastinum, or pulmonary hemorrhage. These, rather than hyaline membrane disease, are the major pulmonary problems in these infants. Because neonatal symptomatic hypoglycemia is commonly found in small-for-dates infants, careful blood glucose monitoring and early feeding are appropriate precautions. Elevated central hematocrit is common in these infants for reasons that are unknown.

80. The answer is E. *(Avery, ed 2. pp 237–239.)* The late anemia of prematurity results from iron deficiency. The premature infant's iron stores depends upon the total body hemoglobin at birth. This is influenced by the infant's size and the circumstances of delivery. The amount of blood withdrawn for laboratory studies and the amount, if any, transfused will affect the timing and the extent of the problem. Iron should be begun when the infant has obtained a weight one and a half times that of birthweight.

81. The answer is C. *(Avery, ed 2. p 1067. Avery and Taeusch, ed 5. pp 901–902.)* Subcutaneous fat necrosis is found in large infants who suffer a long or difficult labor and delivery. Lesions usually appear at about one week of age over cheeks and extensor surfaces. They vary in size, may be colorless or reddish-purple, and feel firm with a sharp border; in addition, they usually produce no symptoms and regress gradually over a period of weeks. Hypercalcemia may be present. The other diagnoses listed in the question have very different clinical appearances.

82. The answer is C. *(Behrman, ed 12. pp 359–360.)* In a difficult delivery in which traction is applied to the head and neck, several injuries, including all those listed in the question, may occur. Erb-Duchenne paralysis affects the fifth and sixth cervical nerves; the affected arm cannot be abducted or externally rotated at the shoulder, and the forearm cannot be flexed or supinated. Injury to the seventh and eighth cervical and first thoracic nerves (Klumpke's paralysis) results in palsy of the hand and also can produce symptoms of Horner's syndrome. Fractures in the upper limb are not associated with a characteristic posture, and passive movement usually elicits pain. Spinal injury causes complete paralysis below the level of injury.

83. The answer is A. *(Avery and Taeusch, ed 5. pp 107–108.)* Infants who are postmature (more than 42 weeks gestation) and show evidence of chronic placental insufficiency (low birth weight for gestational age and wasted appearance, even with good length) have a higher than average chance of being asphyxiated during delivery. Asphyxia leads to the passage of meconium into the amniotic fluid and thus places these infants at risk for meconium aspiration. To prevent or minimize this risk, these infants should have immediate nasopharyngeal suction as their heads are delivered. Immediately after delivery and before initiation of respiration their tracheas must be carefully and thoroughly suctioned through an endotracheal tube under direct vision with a laryngoscope. Afterwards, appropriate and vigorous resuscitative measures should be undertaken to establish adequate ventilation and circulation. Artificial ventilation performed before tracheal suction could well force meconium into smaller airways.

84. The answer is D. *(Fanaroff, ed 3. pp 367–369.)* Periventricular/subependymal hemorrhage is the most common type of intracranial hemorrhage in newborn infants. It occurs in approximately 45 percent of premature infants weighing less than 1500 g. Clinical manifestations occur 24 to 28 hours after a serious hypoxic episode. This type of hemorrhage is not usually catastrophic, and it commonly produces only subtle neurologic deterioration. Systematic symptoms may include an acute drop in hematocrit and arterial P_{O_2} and a marked metabolic acidosis. Serial ultrasound examination of the ventricles and brain are required for diagnosis and proper follow-up.

85. The answer is C. *(Behrman, ed 12. pp 331–335, 1502.)* Turner's syndrome is a genetic disorder characterized by a 45,XO karyotype. At birth affected infants have low weights, short stature, edema over the dorsum of the hands and feet, and loose skin folds at the nape of the neck. Coarse tremulous movements accompanied by ankle clonus; vascular instability as evidenced, for example, by a harlequin color change (a transient, longitudinal division of a body into red and pale halves); softness of parietal bones at the vertex (craniotabes); and a liver that is palpable down to 2 cm below the costal margins – all of these findings often are demonstrated by normal infants and are of no diagnostic significance in the clinical situation presented in the question.

86. The answer is B. *(Fanaroff, ed 3. pp 427–428.)* For the child described in the question, prematurity and the clinical picture presented make the diagnosis of hyaline membrane disease all but inescapable. In this disease lung compliance is reduced to as much as 10 to 20 percent of normal; lung volume also is reduced and as much as a 30 to 60 percent right-to-left shunt of blood may be evident. Some of the shunt may result from a patent ductus arteriosus or foramen ovale, and some may be due to an abnormal ventilation-perfusion ratio in the lung. Minute ventilation is higher than normal and affected infants must work harder in order to sustain adequate breathing.

87. The answer is B. *(Fanaroff, ed 3. pp 432–437.)* Mechanical ventilation improves oxygenation and ventilation by preventing alveolar collapse. Ventilation should be started when arterial P_{O_2} cannot be maintained above 60 mmHg or when P_{CO_2} rises above 55 to 60 mmHg. Because the child's arterial pH is well above 7.25, alkali therapy is not indicated. Elevation of inspired oxygen concentration alone would not affect the hypercarbia.

88. The answer is C. *(Fanaroff, ed 3. pp 430–432.)* Infants whose gestational ages are less than 36 weeks are at risk for retrolental fibroplasia, especially if they are receiving oxygen therapy at an inspired oxygen concentration of greater than 40 percent and if their arterial P_{O_2} is above 80 mmHg. Consequently, for the infant described in the question, the ambient oxygen concentration should be decreased as quickly as possible. This decrease can be best achieved by lowering the concentration slowly and monitoring transcutaneous P_{O_2}. Decreasing the oxygen concentration more radically could provoke the "flip-flop" phenomenon in which arterial P_{O_2} drops farther than expected (when the concentration of inspired oxygen is lowered) and does not return to its previous level when the inspired oxygen is returned to its original higher concentration. Right-to-left shunting may be the cause of the flip-flop.

89. The answer is D. *(Behrman, ed 12. pp 893–894.)* Abdominal distension, choking, the presence of excessive mucus in the oropharynx, and coughing associated with fluid intake all are symptoms of the congenital esophageal anomalies depicted in figures A and D accompanying the question. However, the anomaly illustrated by figure D is the most common and is most likely to produce severe symptoms of regurgitation early in the newborn period; the disorder depicted in figure A usually is diagnosed in older children who have repeated episodes of pneumonitis. The anomaly in figure E is associated with all of the symptoms of anomaly D except abdominal distension, which cannot develop because there is no way for air to enter the gastrointestinal tract. Figures B and C represent the least common anomalies; because the upper esophageal segment is connected directly to the trachea, massive entry of fluid into the lungs can occur.

90. The answer is B. *(Behrman, ed 12. p 1247.)* Failure to give vitamin K prophylactically to newborn infants is associated with a decline in the levels of vitamin K-dependent coagulation factors. In less than 1 percent of infants (but especially those fed human breast milk), the levels reached are low enough to produce hemorrhagic manifestations on the second or third day of life. These manifestations usually include melena, hematuria, and bleeding from the navel; intracranial hemorrhage and hypovolemic shock are serious complications. Diagnosis of this condition is indicated by a prolonged prothrombin time, which reflects inadequate concentrations of factors II, VII, and X in an infant. There is no genetic predisposition to the disease.

91. The answer is C. *(Gellis, ed 11. p 687.)* Newborn infants with localized cyanosis of the face have usually had localized factors such as venous stasis due to an umbilical cord wrapped tightly around the neck or a face presentation operating during the birth process. The peripheral vasoconstriction associated with cold stress can affect the face, and this is even more noticeable when the face is myxedematous from hypothyroidism. An unusual but important cause of cyanosis above the neck is obstruction of the superior vena cava. Dusky or cyanotic episodes at any age often indicate serious disease and must not be ignored.

92. The answer is A. *(Fanaroff, ed 3. pp 154–156.)* The effect of a drug on the fetus is determined not only by the nature of the drug but also by the timing and degree of exposure in utero. Heparin does not cross the placental barrier and cannot directly affect the fetus once pregnancy is well established. Hydantoin may cause birth defects when given to some individuals during the first trimester. Penicillin and aluminum hydroxide have not been found to affect the fetus. Propanalol, which may also cause growth retardation when given throughout pregnancy, diminishes the ability of an asphyxiated infant to respond by increasing heart rate and cardiac output. It has also been associated with hypoglycemia.

93. The answer is D. *(Avery, ed 2. pp 812–813.)* The finding of hydramnios can signal the presence in a neonate of high intestinal obstruction, signs of which include abdominal distension and early and repeated regurgitation of intestinal contents. Distension may not be present if the obstruction is very high or if the constant vomiting keeps the intestine decompressed. Because the presence of bile-stained fluid in the vomitus of the infant described in the question places the possible obstruction distal to the ampulla of Vater, esophageal atresia and pyloric stenosis are ruled out. The "double bubble" sign on the accompanying x-ray is characteristic of duodenal atresia, which also is compatible with the infant's history. Midgut volvulus, which usually obstructs the bowel in the area of the duodenojejunal junction, most often produces signs after an affected infant is three or four days old; in addition, several loops of small bowel are typically seen on x-ray. Gastric duplication does not usually produce intestinal obstruction; a cystic mass may be palpated on abdominal examination.

94. The answer is D. *(Kliegman, N Engl J Med 310:1099–1100.)* If the diagnosis in a neonate of necrotizing enterocolitis either is strongly entertained or is confirmed by finding pneumatosis intestinalis on abdominal x-ray, therapy should consist of gastric drainage, discontinuance of oral feedings, administration of oral and systemic antibiotics, and vigorous administration of intravenous fluids that include vascular volume expanders, as needed, and as high a caloric content as possible. Because bowel perforation, a serious complication, occurs frequently, signs of acute deterioration must be watched for very carefully. Only if intestinal infarction or perforation is believed to be present is surgical intervention generally advocated. Steroids are not a recommended treatment for this disease.

95. The answer is B. *(Kliegman, N Engl J Med 310:1093–1094.)* The early clinical signs of neonatal necrotizing enterocolitis include gastric distension, retention of gastric contents between feedings, and the passage of blood-streaked stools. This disorder usually occurs in premature infants who, because of cardiovascular shock or hypoxia (often associated with severe hyaline membrane disease), have had their blood supply preferentially shunted away from the gut to the heart and brain. Intestinal ischemia and invasion of affected bowel by enteric flora are thought to be the two major pathogenetic processes involved in necrotizing enterocolitis. Hypertonic feeding is believed to play a role. No relationship exists between necrotizing enterocolitis and the meconium plug syndrome, calcium, therapy, or maternal bowel disease.

96. The answer is D. *(Behrman, ed 12. pp 881–882.)* The infant pictured in the question has an obvious bilateral cleft lip and palate. This defect occurs in 4 to 7 percent of the siblings of affected infants; its incidence in the general population, on the other hand, is 1 in 1000. Although affected infants are likely to have feeding problems initially, these problems usually can be overcome by feeding in a propped-up position and using special nipples. Complications include recurrent otitis media and hearing loss as well as speech defects, which may be present in spite of good anatomic closure. Repair of a cleft lip usually is performed within the first two months of life; the palate is repaired later, usually between the ages of six months and five years.

97. The answer is A. *(American Academy of Pediatrics, p 187.)* The pregnancy of the woman described in the question is considered high-risk by virtue of her history of abortions and the premature onset of labor. The woman's infant will very likely require neonatal intensive care. Statistics show that the mortality rate for low-birth-weight infants is lowest if they are born in centers having facilities for prenatal intensive care (one-third of all deaths of premature infants occur within 24 hours of birth). For this reason, and because a mother's womb is thought to be the best "transport incubator" available, the woman described should be transferred to the referral perinatal center immediately (i.e., before the birth of her child).

98. The answer is B. *(Avery, ed 2. pp 295–297.)* Glucose loading of the mother will result in fetal hyperglycemia, which causes insulin release and reactive hypoglycemia. Careful medical support of the antepartum woman diminishes the hypertrophy of the fetal eyelet cells. Careful monitoring of the infant with proper intravenous infusion of glucose in amounts 100 to 105 percent of the requirements of a normal infant can usually prevent hypoglycemia. A neutral thermal environment diminishes glucose consumption and, therefore, helps with glucose homeostasis.

99. The answer is D. *(Avery and Taeusch, ed 5. pp 437–439.)* Nearly three-fourths of abdominal masses in newborn infants involve and stem from the kidney. In the infant described in the question, the presence both of a mass in the flank and of gross hematuria further indicates a renal lesion. A mass discovered at 20 hours of age suggests sudden enlargement of a kidney; this finding makes the diagnosis of renal vein thrombosis most likely in the infant described. Also in support of this diagnosis are the child's pallor and clinical illness and the fact that the mother is diabetic. Evaluation of the infant should include an intravenous pyleogram, coagulation studies, and measurement of the serum creatinine, blood gases, urea nitrogen, and electrolytes.

100. The answer is B (1, 3). *(Behrman, ed 12. p 382.)* The presence of anemia must not be overlooked in infants who have hemolytic disease and are being treated for hyperbilirubinemia with, for example, phototherapy. Once phototherapy is started, the skin color of affected infants can no longer be relied upon in an assessment of either jaundice or pallor; similarly, scleral icterus is an unreliable indicator of the degree of hyperbilirubinemia.

101. The answer is B (1, 3). *(Fanaroff, ed 3. pp 374–377.)* Because of active transport, calcium stores accumulate in a fetus during the third trimester regardless of the maternal nutritional state. Breast-fed infants have higher calcium and lower phosphorus levels than bottle-fed infants due to the higher calcium:phosphorus ratio in breast milk as compared to cow's milk. Stress associated with asphyxia or a difficult labor or delivery may cause elevations in calcitonin and glucocorticoids, which in turn may cause symptomatic hypocalcemia. The incidence of hypocalcemia is higher than normal among premature infants and infants of diabetic mothers due to immaturity of the parathyroid.

102. The answer is B (1, 3). *(Behrman, ed 12. pp 149–151.)* Human breast milk is fresh, sterile, and always at the right temperature. It is easily digestible, is associated with fewer gastrointestinal disturbances than cow's milk, produces no allergic manifestations, and contains several factors, including antibodies, that are believed to provide protection from infection. However, breast-feeding is associated with a higher incidence of physiologic jaundice than bottle-feeding. Usually cessation of breast-feeding is not necessary. A brief cessation of breast-feeding is almost always the only treatment necessary. No significant difference in emotional well-being appears to exist between well-nurtured breast-fed and bottle-fed infants.

103. The answer is E (all). *(Fanaroff, ed 3. pp 764–765.)* Factors that reduce the amount of unconjugated bilirubin bound to albumin (and therefore cause an increase in free unconjugated bilirubin) increase the risk of kernicterus. Among these factors are the following: hypoalbuminemia; acidosis, which decreases the affinity of bulirubin for albumin; and certain drugs (e.g., salicylates and sulfonamides) and other compounds (such as nonesterified fatty acids, which are elevated during cold stress) that as anions compete with bilirubin for albumin binding sites. Acidosis and hypoxia also are believed to increase brain-cell susceptibility to bilirubin toxicity.

104. The answer is A (1, 2, 3). *(Avery and Taeusch, ed 5. pp 654–655.)* Normal term neonates demonstrate a large number of reflex patterns that are mediated by the brainstem or spinal cord. These reactions include the Moro (startle) reflex; the sucking and rooting reflexes; the stepping reflex, by which movements of forward progression are elicited on a flat surface; the placing reflex, which produces leg flexion; and the palmar and plantar grasps, which result from slight pressure on the palms and soles. The parachute reaction, which is extension of the arms and hands that occur when an infant in the prone position is brought sharply toward a firm surface, does not appear until the age of nine months.

105. The answer is C (2, 4). *(Avery, ed 2. pp 209–213.)* Infants born at 33 weeks gestation are covered with vernix and have smooth skin and fine wooly hair. They have no breast tissue, and because ear cartilage is scant, ears recoil slowly when folded. There are one or two anterior sole creases, and in the female the clitoris is readily visible between widely separated labia majora. At rest, the arms are extended and the hips flexed. There is some resistance in bringing the heel to the ear, and the elbow passes the midline but does not reach to the opposite shoulder. Although sucking, rooting, and the grasp and Moro reflexes are all present, they are not fully developed.

106. The answer is E (all). *(Behrman, ed 12. pp 394–395.)* Infants born to narcotic addicts are more likely than other children to exhibit a variety of problems, including perinatal complications, prematurity, and low birth weight. The onset of withdrawal symptoms commonly occurs during an infant's first two days of life. The most characteristic symptoms in these infants are hyperirritability and coarse tremors. Other symptoms include vomiting, diarrhea, fever, high-pitched cry, and hyperventilation; seizures, respiratory depression, and other symptoms are less common.

107. The answer is E (all). *(Fanaroff, ed 3. pp 240–250.)* Studies in the last ten years have shown several benefits of early close contact between mothers and their newborn infants. The mothers show more affectionate behavior toward their infants and use more descriptive words and questions when talking to them than mothers who have less or late contact with their infants. In the early close contact group there were fewer mothering disorders including child abuse, neglect, and abandonment. The infants smiled more, responded to their mothers' voices, and cried less. Breast-feeding was also prolonged in close early contact group.

108. The answer is A (1, 2, 3). *(Avery, ed 2. p 631.)* Phenylketonuria is an auto-somal recessive disease that leads to mental and motor retardation in untreated infants. Affected infants appear normal during the perinatal period; clinical signs of the retardation of brain development may first appear at the age of four months. The primary defect is an inability to synthesize tyrosine from phenylalanine, which, as a result, accumulates in the urine by older children but not neonates. When the plasma phenylalanine level is 20 mg/100 ml or higher, dietary restriction of this amino acid is indicated.

109. The answer is B (1, 3). *(Gellis, ed 11. p 687.)* On the skull of a newborn infant, a swelling that is sharply demarcated by the margins of one particular bone typically indicates a cephalhematoma. It is reported in 1.5 to 2.5 percent of births, especially those associated with obstetric difficulty at the outlet. Systematic study has shown that 5.4 percent of cephalehematomas are accompanied by a linear skull fracture. The majority of these swellings resorb spontaneously within a few weeks; a few, however, become calcified and persist for a few months as prominent lumps on the head. No treatment is needed in either event. Needle aspiration is contraindicated because of the possibility of introducing infection. The injury occurs during the delivery process. Rarely is the lesion noticeable before the second day.

110. The answer is B (1, 3). *(Avery and Taeusch, ed 5. pp 909–914.)* Although retinopathy of prematurity has been described in term infants, most infants after 34 weeks gestation will have retinas developed enough so that involvement, if any, is minimal. Mild degrees of this condition may be manifest as myopia. The condition, once thought to be caused by over-treatment with oxygen, is now found mostly in very immature infants of less than 30 weeks gestation who require ventilatory support. Retinopathy of prematurity best correlates with immaturity and with serious illness rather than with P_{O_2} levels. Vitamin E may play a role in preventing the scarring. It does not affect the development of the proliferative phase which occurs (and spontaneously regresses) in a high percentage of the very premature infants.

111. The answer is D (4). *(Fanaroff, ed 3. pp 469–476. Hallman, Pediatr Clin North Am 29:1057–1075, 1982. Phelps, Pediatr Clin North Am 29:1233–1240, 1982.)* Bronchopulmonary dysplasia (BPD) typically occurs in premature infants, usually in association with oxygen administered by assisted positive pressure ventillation. It is characterized by a prolonged requirement for oxygen with pulmonary edema followed by pulmonary fibrosis and a "bubbly" or cystic appearance to the lungs on chest x-ray. Although neonatal lung diseases such as hyaline membrane disease and meconium aspiration, which require therapy with oxygen given by positive pressure, may be followed by BPD, these diseases do not appear to be etiologic and do not tend to lead to BPD in the full-term infant. The possible roles of direct oxygen toxicity and of pressure damage are not fully understood, particularly because extreme prematurity may be followed by BPD in the absence of oxygen therapy. Vitamin E has not yet been proven to prevent BPD.

112. The answer is B (1, 3). *(Fanaroff, ed 3. pp 854–858.)* Infants of diabetic mothers have a very rapid drop in blood glucose levels after delivery and are often hypoglycemic within six hours of birth. Hyperinsulinism, either alone or in combination with diminished epinephrine and glucagon responses, is believed to be the major cause of the hypoglycemia, macrosomia, and other metabolic abnormalities seen in these infants. Hypoglycemia in infants of diabetic mothers is less frequently symptomatic than in small-for-dates infants. Hypoglycemia is best prevented by frequent blood sugar monitoring and early feeding of affected infants. If necessary, a constant intravenous infusion of a 10% to 15% glucose solution may be given. Rapid infusion of glucose at high concentrations may result in rebound hypoglycemia after initial hyperglycemia.

113. The answer is A (1, 2, 3). *(Behrman, ed 12. pp 377–378.)* Meconium ileus occurs among newborn infants who have cystic fibrosis, because the absence in these infants of normal pancreatic enzymes makes their meconium abnormally tenacious. Affected neonates present with signs of intestinal obstruction, and numerous, doughy masses of intestine are palpable throughout the abdomen; no discoloration of the abdominal wall occurs. Plain films of the abdomen characteristically show unevenly dilated loops of bowel that, because of a mixture of meconium and air, appear granular. Meconium ileus is often fatal.

114. The answer is A (1, 2, 3). *(Fanaroff, ed 3. pp 562–563.)* Apnea is common in premature infants but is distinctly unusual in the term baby. When it occurs there is almost always an identifiable cause. Sepsis, congenital heart disease, and seizures are recognized causes of apnea in term newborns and may not be evident until several days after birth. Hypoglycemia not associated with other illness is also a cause of apnea but would be very unusual as late as the third day in a term newborn.

115. The answer is A (1, 2, 3). *(Fanaroff, ed 3. p 714.)* Twin-to-twin transfusions occur in about 15 percent of monochorionic twins and commonly causes intrauterine death. This disorder should be suspected when the hematocrits of twins differ by more than 15 percent units (e.g., 45 percent and 61 percent). The donor twin is likely to have oligohydramnios, anemia, and hypovolemia with evidence of shock; the recipient twin is likely to have hydramnios and plethora and to be larger than the donor twin. As the central venous hematocrit rises above 65 percent, blood viscosity increases exponentially, putting affected infants at risk for several complications, including respiratory distress, hyperbilirubinemia, hypoglycemia, hypocalcemia, renal vein thrombosis, cyanosis, congestive heart failure, and convulsions.

116. The answer is C (2, 4). *(Behrman, ed 12. p 342.)* Twin pregnancies are associated with fourfold increase in perinatal mortality as compared to single pregnancies; this increase is particularly notable among monochorionic twins. As a rule, the mortality rate is the same for first- and second-born twins. Twins are likely to be born prematurely, and if born after 35 weeks gestation, they are likely to be small for dates. Monoamniotic twins have an increased incidence of asphyxia because of the greater likelihood of cord entanglement. Twin pregnancies also have an increased incidence of severe congenital malformations, bleeding during labor, and twin-to-twin transfusions as well as maternal complications.

117. The answer is A (1, 2, 3). *(Behrman, ed 12. pp 988–990.)* Severe respiratory distress that is present from birth in an infant who has a scaphoid abdomen suggests the presence of a diaphragmatic hernia. Breath sounds are absent on the affected side of the chest, and the heart sounds are displaced to the unaffected side. A chest x-ray showing intestinal loops in the chest (usually on the left side) and displacement of the mediastinum to the unaffected side is diagnostic of diaphragmatic hernia. Definitive treatment is surgical and must be carried out on an emergency basis. Before surgery, however, affected infants must be resuscitated as effectively as possible. A nasogastric tube with intermittent suction should be placed to minimize the accumulation of air in the herniated intestine. If positive pressure ventilation is required, it should be used with caution in order to avoid a pneumothorax in lungs that are being unevenly ventilated. Metabolic acidosis should be corrected promptly.

118–121. The answers are: 118-C, 119-A, 120-B, 121-B. *(Smith, ed 3. pp 182–183.)* Sporadic aniridia is found in 1 to 2 percent of children with Wilms' tumor. Genitourinary anomalies and hemihypertrophy are associated with this tumor in 13 percent of patients.

Waardenburg's syndrome is inherited as an autosomal dominant trait with variable penetrance. It includes, in decreasing order of frequency, the following anomalies: lateral displacement of the medial canthi; broad nasal bridge; medial hyperplasia of the eyebrows; partial albinism commonly expressed by a white forelock or heterochromia (or both); and deafness in 20 percent of cases.

A flat capillary hemangioma in the distribution of the trigeminal nerve is the basic lesion in the Sturge-Weber syndrome. The malformation also involves the meninges and results in anoxic damage to the underlying cerebral cortex. The damage is manifested clinically to grand mal seizures, mental deficiency, and hemiparesis or hemianopia on the contralateral side. The etiology is unknown.

Infants who have tuberous sclerosis often are born with hypopigmented oval or irregularly shaped skin macules. Cerebral sclerotic tubers are also present from birth and become visible radiographically during the second year of life. Myoclonic seizures, present in infancy, may convert to grand mal seizures later in childhood. Adenoma sebaceum appears at two to five years of age. The disease, which also affects the eyes, kidneys, heart, bones, and lungs, is inherited as an autosomal dominant trait with variable expression; new mutations are very common.

122–125. The answers are: 122-B, 123-C, 124-E, 125-A. *(Behrman, ed 12. pp 378–381.)* In premature infants who have physiologic jaundice (curve B), serum bilirubin levels reach a peak of 8 to 12 mg/100 ml at five to seven days of age; jaundice disappears after the tenth day of life. Physiologic jaundice in full-term neonates (curve D), on the other hand, appears at two to three days of age; peak bilirubin levels of about 5 to 6 mg/100 ml appear at two to four days of age. Bilirubin levels drop below 2 mg/100 ml within a few days.

Jaundice in infants who have hypothyroidism (curve E) initially appears to be physiologic. However, jaundice associated with these infants (as well as infants who have pyloric stenosis) can persist for several weeks.

In neonates born with erythroblastosis fetalis (curve A), jaundice is apparent in the first 24 hours of life. Bilirubin accumulates rapidly, reaching a peak level (up to 20 mg/100 ml) that varies with the degree of hemolysis. The duration of jaundice is also dependent on the severity of the disease.

Curve C on the graph presented is compatible with a diagnosis of septicemia. In this disorder jaundice appears between the fourth and seventh days of life; as the infection is treated, bilirubin levels return to normal.

The Cardiovascular System

Harvey L. Chernoff

DIRECTIONS: Each question below contains five suggested answers. Choose the **one** best response to each question.

126. In an infant the major clinical manifestation of digitalis toxicity would be

(A) headache
(B) dizziness
(C) vomiting
(D) visual disturbances
(E) anorexia

127. A 15-year-old girl of short stature who has neck webbing and sexual infantilism is found to have coarctation of the aorta. The most likely diagnosis is

(A) Marfan's syndrome
(B) Down's syndrome
(C) Turner's syndrome
(D) Ellis-van Creveld syndrome
(E) an unrelated group of findings

128. Electrocardiography of a cyanotic two-day-old infant shows a suggestion of right ventricular enlargement. The child's chest x-ray is presented below. The most likely diagnosis is

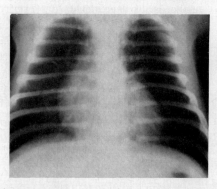

(A) tetralogy of Fallot
(B) transposition of the great vessels
(C) tricuspid atresia
(D) pulmonic valve atresia
(E) Ebstein's anomaly

129. The incidence of congenital heart disease in the offspring of mothers with congenital heart disease is

(A) 1 percent
(B) 1 to 4 percent
(C) 3 to 12 percent
(D) 14 percent
(E) 23 percent

130. A male infant presents at age two days with a harsh grade 3/6 pansystolic murmur in the third and fourth space along the left sternal border with radiation to the apex. The murmur sounds louder by one grade the next day and is associated with a thrill. The findings remain unchanged until day four when he develops a diastolic grade II/VI rumble over the apex in addition to the pansystolic murmur and thrill. These findings point to a diagnosis of

(A) ventricular septal defect
(B) ventricular septal defect and aortic regurgitation
(C) atrial septal defect
(D) atrial septal defect and pulmonary regurgitation
(E) none of the above

131. A two-day-old infant is in congestive heart failure. Cardiac catheterization and angiography reveal a hypoplastic left ventricle and aortic atresia. Which of the following statements about this child is true?

(A) Aortic valvuloplasty, if performed early, will be of help
(B) The child's condition should improve dramatically with treatment of the congestive heart failure
(C) Digitalization should be an effective medical treatment
(D) The child is unlikely to benefit from surgery
(E) The average survival time of infants like the one described is two months

132. Pulmonary vascular resistance in an infant begins to diminish rapidly following delivery. This physiologic change is thought to be regulated primarily by

(A) a rise in arterial P_{O_2}
(B) a decrease in intrathoracic pressure
(C) a reduction in the tortuosity of the pulmonary vasculature
(D) closure of the ductus arteriosus
(E) release of humoral factors after cessation of placental circulation

133. A three-day-old infant has developed tachypnea and tachycardia. Initial examination shows hepatomegaly, cardiomegaly, and peripheral pulses present in the upper extremities and the femoral arteries. A few hours later, however, the pulses in the femoral arteries have disappeared. The infant is minimally cyanotic. The most likely diagnosis is congestive heart failure, patent ductus arteriosus, and

(A) postductal aortic coarctation
(B) preductal aortic coarctation
(C) ventricular septal defect
(D) tetralogy of Fallot
(E) none of the above

134. A child presents with tall stature, long fingers and toes, and scoliosis. Cardiac examination would be most likely to demonstrate

(A) aortic stenosis
(B) mitral stenosis
(C) mitral regurgitation
(D) pulmonary incompetence
(E) none of the above

135. A three-month-old infant has a history of short episodes during feeding of apparent abdominal pain associated with diaphoresis, duskiness, and rapid pulse and breathing. A pansystolic murmur that was not present when the child was examined two months earlier is heard over the cardiac apex. Which of the following studies would be most likely to aid in reaching the correct diagnosis?

(A) Chest x-ray
(B) Angiocardiography
(C) Electrocardiography
(D) Phonocardiography
(E) Dye dilution study

136. An eight-month-old infant has a one-week history of increasing shortness of breath and fatigue. Examination of the infant reveals evidence of severe congestive heart failure; radiography of the chest shows marked cardiomegaly, and electrocardiography reveals left ventricular hypertrophy with negative T waves in the left chest leads. No other physical abnormalities are noted.
The most likely diagnosis for this child is

(A) an aberrant left coronary artery
(B) idiopathic hypertrophic subaortic stenosis
(C) Pompe's disease (glycogen storage disease, type II)
(D) acute myocarditis
(E) endocardial fibroelastosis

137. A two-year-old boy is brought into the emergency room with a complaint of fever for six days and development of a limp. On examination he is found to have mild erythematous macular exanthem over his body, ocular conjunctivitis, dry, cracked lips, a red throat, and considerable cervical lymphadenopathy. The skin around his nails is peeling. There is a grade II/VI vibratory systolic ejection murmur at the lower left sternal border. He refuses to bear weight on his left leg. On questioning, his mother relates that a cousin who visited a week earlier had been taking penicillin for a sore throat. A white blood cell count and differential show predominantly neutrophils with increased platelets on smear and a sedimentation rate of 100 mm.

The most likely diagnosis of this boy's condition is

(A) scarlet fever
(B) rheumatic fever
(C) Kawasaki disease
(D) juvenile rheumatoid arthritis
(E) infectious mononucleosis

138. An ill-appearing two-week-old girl is brought to the emergency room. She is pale and dyspneic with a respiratory rate of 80/minute. Heart rate is 195/minute, sounds are distant, and there is a suggestion of a gallop. There is cardiomegaly by x-ray. An echocardiogram demonstrates poor ventricular function, dilated ventricles and, possibly, dilation of the left atrium. Electrocardiogram shows ventricular depolarization complexes that have low voltage. Initial administration of diuretics and continued use of digoxin brings about progressive improvement over about three days. The diagnosis suggested by this clinical picture is

(A) myocarditis
(B) endocardial fibroelastosis
(C) pericarditis
(D) aberrant left coronary artery arising from pulmonary artery
(E) glycogen storage disease of the heart

139. A newborn infant has a history of occasional cyanosis. On examination, a grade III/VI harsh pansystolic (holosystolic) murmur is heard along the lower left sternal border. Radiography of the chest shows a normal cardiothoracic ratio, normal pulmonary vascular markings, and a right aortic arch. The most likely diagnosis is

(A) a ventricular septal defect
(B) a ventricular septal defect and transportation of the great vessels
(C) tetralogy of Fallot
(D) truncus arteriosus
(E) anomalous pulmonary venous return

140. Of the combined ventricular output of a normal fetal heart, the placenta receives about 45 percent and the fetal lungs only about 8 percent. This distribution is determined primarily by which of the following factors in a fetus?

(A) P_{O_2}
(B) P_{CO_2}
(C) pH
(D) Blood pressure
(E) Vascular resistance

141. A neonate born at term presents in the first day of life with cyanosis and progressive dyspnea. A chest x-ray reveals a heart of normal size but a significant increase in pulmonary vascular and interstitial markings. This infant most likely is suffering from

(A) transposition of the great vessels
(B) infracardiac total anomalous pulmonary venous return
(C) pulmonic atresia
(D) hyaline membrane disease
(E) mitral stenosis

142. Individuals who have chronic hypoxia have an increased hematocrit. Although the precise metabolic pathways are not yet clear, most authorities attribute the stimulation of red blood cell production to release of erythropoietin by the

(A) spleen
(B) liver
(C) kidneys
(D) bone marrow
(E) lungs

143. A newborn infant has mild cyanosis, diaphoresis, poor peripheral pulses, hepatomegaly, and cardiomegaly. Respiratory rate is 60 per minute, and heart rate is 230 per minute. The child most likely has congestive heart failure due to

(A) a large atrial septal defect and valvular pulmonic stenosis
(B) a ventricular septal defect and transposition of the great vessels
(C) atrial flutter and partial atrioventricular block
(D) hypoplastic left heart syndrome
(E) paroxysmal atrial tachycardia

144. A three-year-old child has had two episodes of syncope. On examination, blood pressure is normal in the arms and legs; no murmurs are heard. Prior neurologic evaluation revealed no neurologic abnormalities. The study most likely to aid in diagnosing this child's condition would be

(A) electrocardiography
(B) vectorcardiography
(C) echocardiography
(D) isotope aniography
(E) cardiac catheterization

145. The most common congenital heart lesion is

(A) pulmonic stenosis
(B) patent ductus arteriosus
(C) atrial septal defect
(D) ventricular septal defect
(E) tetralogy of Fallot

146. A five-year-old boy presents with a grade V/VI harsh ejection systolic murmur in the second interspace at the right sternal border. The murmur radiates to the neck and upper left sternal border. The right brachial pulse is brisk, the left diminished. Blood pressures are right arm 110/60 mmHg, left arm 100/60 mmHg, and right leg 120/60 mmHg. He has a small chin, full lips, open mouth, upturned nose, and wide-set eyes. An electrocardiogram shows left ventricular hypertrophy. The most likely defect would be

(A) bicuspid aortic valve
(B) valvular aortic stenosis
(C) discrete subvalvular aortic stenosis
(D) supravalvular aortic stenosis
(E) aortic coarctation

147. Congestive heart failure due to congenital heart disease is encountered most frequently in which of the following age groups?

(A) Less than six months of age
(B) Six to twelve months of age
(C) One to five years of age
(D) Six to fifteen years of age
(E) Sixteen to twenty-one years of age

148. A child with an atrial septal defect has an accentuated pulmonic closure sound; electrocardiography shows right ventricular hypertrophy. These findings suggest that the child most likely has

(A) valvular pulmonic stenosis
(B) infundibular pulmonic stenosis
(C) pulmonary hypertension
(D) congestive heart failure
(E) pulmonic regurgitation

149. A two-year-old child with minimal cyanosis has a quadruple rhythm, a systolic ejection murmur in the pulmonic area, and a pansystolic murmur along the lower left sternal border. An electrocardiogram is obtained and shows P pulmonale and a ventricular block pattern in the right chest leads. The child most likely has

(A) tricuspid regurgitation and pulmonic stenosis
(B) pulmonic stenosis and a ventricular septal defect (tetralogy of Fallot)
(C) an atrioventricular canal
(D) Ebstein's anomaly
(E) Wolff-Parkinson-White syndrome

150. The major electrocardiographic abnormality in children who have ostium primum atrial septal defects (endocardial cushion defects) is

(A) right axis deviation
(B) left axis deviation
(C) incomplete right bundle-branch block
(D) first-degree atrioventricular block
(E) second-degree atrioventricular block

151. A four-year-old girl is brought to the pediatrician's office. Her father reports that she suddenly became pale and stopped running while he had been playfully chasing her. During play she had been very excited, laughing to the point at which "she almost lost her breath." After 30 minutes, she was no longer pale and wanted to resume the game. She has never had a previous episode nor ever been cyanotic. Her physical examination was normal as were her chest x-ray and echocardiogram. An electrocardiogram showed the patterns seen in figures A and B below. The most likely cause of the episode is

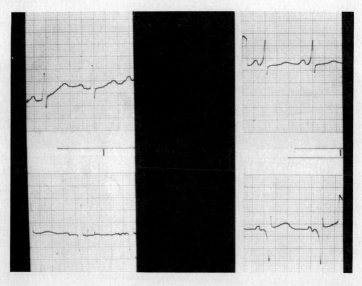

(A) paroxysmal ventricular tachycardia
(B) paroxysmal supraventricular tachycardia
(C) Wolff-Parkinson-White syndrome
(D) an unsuspected congenital heart defect
(E) excessive stress during play

152. Examination of a newborn infant reveals a heart rate of 60 beats per minute. At no time during the next three days does the rate rise above 68 beats per minute. Electrocardiography would be most likely to demonstrate

(A) second-degree atrioventricular block
(B) complete atrioventricular block
(C) complete atrioventricular block and atrial fibrillation
(D) sinus arrest with an idioventricular rhythm
(E) sinus bradycardia

153. A child has a history of spiking fevers, which have been as high as 40°C (104°F). She has spindle-shaped swelling of finger joints and complains of upper sternal pain. She had streptococcal pharyngitis two weeks before her fevers began. The most likely diagnosis is

(A) rheumatic fever
(B) rheumatoid arthritis
(C) toxic synovitis
(D) septic arthritis
(E) osteoarthritis

154. A three-day-old infant has had progressively deepening cyanosis since birth but no respiratory distress. Chest radiography demonstrates no cardiomegaly and normal pulmonary vasculature. An electrocardiogram shows an axis of 120 degrees and right ventricular prominence. The congenital cardiac malformation most likely responsible for the cyanosis is

(A) tetralogy of Fallot
(B) transposition of the great vessels
(C) tricuspid atresia
(D) total anomalous pulmonary venous return below the diaphragm
(E) pulmonary atresia with intact ventricular septum

155. The presence of endocardial cushion defects is most likely to be associated with

(A) Turner's syndrome
(B) Noonan's syndrome
(C) Down's syndrome
(D) Marfan's syndrome
(E) Hunter-Hurler syndrome

156. A four-year-old child presents with a grade III/VI ejection systolic murmur over the pulmonic area. The pulmonic component of the second sound is accentuated. Electrocardiography reveals right ventricular hypertrophy, and chest x-rays show normal pulmonary vascular markings with mild prominence of the pulmonary artery segment. The most likely diagnosis is

(A) atrial septal defect
(B) partial anomalous pulmonary venous return
(C) valvular pulmonic stenosis
(D) supravalvular pulmonic stenosis
(E) none of the above

DIRECTIONS: Each question below contains four suggested answers of which **one or more** is correct. Choose the answer:

A	if	**1, 2, and 3**	are correct
B	if	**1 and 3**	are correct
C	if	**2 and 4**	are correct
D	if	**4**	is correct
E	if	**1, 2, 3, and 4**	are correct

157. A newborn infant who is in respiratory distress because of congestive heart failure would be likely to exhibit which of the following breathing patterns?

(1) Tachypnea
(2) Grunting
(3) Hyperpnea
(4) Periodic breathing

158. The blood pressure elevation seen in children as they advance into the teenage years is a function of

(1) progressive increase in cardiac output
(2) normally increasing hematocrit and resulting increase in viscosity
(3) hyperkinetic circulatory state
(4) progressive increase in peripheral vascular resistance

159. The hypoplastic left-heart syndrome describes a group of left-sided lesions that can result in underdevelopment of the left ventricle. Among these left-sided lesions may be included

(1) aortic atresia
(2) hypoplasia of the aortic arch
(3) mitral atresia
(4) endocardial fibroelastosis

160. A newborn infant weighing 2000 g (4 lb, 6 oz) presents with cyanosis; there is no evidence of respiratory distress. Cardiac catheterization reveals pulmonic valve atresia and pulmonary flow that derives from the aorta through a patent ductus arteriosus. Maintenance of adequate pulmonary blood flow may be achieved by

(1) aorticopulmonary anastomosis
(2) administration of E-type prostaglandins
(3) formalin infiltration of the ductus arteriosus
(4) pulmonary valvotomy

161. At birth the transition from fetal to extrauterine circulation is associated with a rapid decrease in pulmonary arterial resistance due to

(1) increased oxygen tension producing pulmonary arterial vasodilation
(2) increased oxygen tension stimulating closure of the ductus arteriosus
(3) initial inspiration producing inflation of the lungs
(4) closure of the foramen ovale, producing increased right heart and, therefore, pulmonary arterial blood volume

---

SUMMARY OF DIRECTIONS

A	B	C	D	E
1,2,3 only	1,3 only	2,4 only	4 only	All are correct

---

162. A newborn infant of a diabetic mother presents with signs of congestive heart failure. Laboratory analysis is likely to reveal

(1) hypoglycemia
(2) hyperbilirubinemia
(3) hypocalcemia
(4) anemia

163. Which of the following manifestations of acute rheumatic fever can be relieved by salicylate or steroid therapy?

(1) Carditis
(2) Abdominal pain
(3) Arthritis
(4) Chorea

164. An eight-year-old boy is brought into the hospital with a complaint of a seizure which occurred while chasing a friend. There is a history of recent onset of fatigue and heavier breathing than peers during play. On examination he is thin, in no distress, and without cyanosis, clubbing, edema, thrills, or murmurs. The pulmonic second sound is mildly accentuated. Neurologic examination reveals no abnormalities except for a mild hearing deficit. Further evaluation should be directed toward ruling out the possibility of

(1) long Q-T syndrome
(2) aortic stenosis
(3) primary pulmonary hypertension
(4) paroxysmal atrial tachycardia

165. A cyanotic 20-month-old child has a continuous murmur over the precordium and over the back. The child is in no visible distress. This clinical picture can be associated with which of the following disorders?

(1) Truncus arteriosus
(2) Total anomalous pulmonary venous return
(3) Tetralogy of Fallot
(4) Patent ductus arteriosus

166. Which of the following lesions, when combined with a ventricular septal defect, frequently can cause cardiac decompensation in newborn infants?

(1) Preductal aortic coarctation
(2) Postductal aortic coarctation
(3) Patent ductus arteriosus
(4) Tetralogy of Fallot

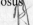

167. A three-year-old boy, who otherwise appears well, presents with a history of pallor and a heart rate that has been persistently rapid for the last 30 minutes. Examination reveals a pansystolic murmur along the lower left sternal border and at the apex. Electrocardiography shows a sinus arrhythmia at a rate of 100 beats per minute, a QR pattern in V_1 with no right bundle-branch block, and a pure R wave in V_6; the PR interval is questionably prolonged.

These findings may be associated with

(1) atrioventricularis communis
(2) Ebstein's anomaly
(3) an ostium primum atrial septal defect
(4) corrected transposition of the great vessels

168. Mitral valve surgery for regurgitation presents difficult problems in that these valves are crucial to the functioning of the left ventricle. In children the problem is compounded since most mitral valve regurgitation is due to marked abnormality of the valve leaflets and chordae tendinae in association with defects of the atrial and ventricular septa leading to severe symptoms presenting in infancy. The best results can be achieved by

(1) homograft valve replacement
(2) medical management
(3) Coumadin
(4) mitral valve repair

169. The performance of an atrial septostomy during cardiac catheterization may be helpful in patients with which of the following?

(1) Tricuspid atresia with hypoplastic right ventricle
(2) Tricuspid atresia with ventricular septal defect
(3) Tricuspid atresia with severe pulmonic stenosis
(4) Tricuspid atresia with transposition of the great arteries

170. Cardiac catheterization shows that a child has a partial anomalous pulmonary venous return to the right atrium with an intact atrial septum. Pulmonary artery and right ventricular pressures are not elevated. Physical examination might be expected to reveal

(1) pulmonic ejection systolic murmur
(2) fixed wide splitting of the second heart sound
(3) right ventricular heave
(4) accentuated pulmonic valve closure sound (P_2)

171. Surgical treatment of premature infants with patent ductus arteriosus refractory to medical treatment results in

(1) high hospital survival
(2) reduced incidence of necrotizing enterocolitis
(3) earlier endotracheal extubation
(4) increased morbidity and mortality

172. Maldevelopment of the endocardial cushions may result in

(1) an atrial septal defect
(2) a ventricular septal defect
(3) deformity of the mitral valve
(4) deformity of the tricuspid valve

SUMMARY OF DIRECTIONS

A	B	C	D	E
1,2,3 only	1,3 only	2,4 only	4 only	All are correct

173. A child who has known valvular pulmonic stenosis (i.e., a pulmonic ejection click and a stenotic systolic murmur) has had increasing narrowing of the pulmonic valve. Auscultatory evidence of this narrowing could include

(1) earlier appearance of the ejection click
(2) increased intensity of the systolic murmur
(3) extension of the systolic murmur beyond the aortic component
(4) increased intensity of the ejection click

DIRECTIONS: The group of questions below consists of lettered choices followed by several numbered items. For each numbered item select the **one** lettered choice with which it is **most** closely associated. Each lettered choice may be used once, more than once, or not at all.

Questions 174–176.

For each set of findings select the diagnosis with which it is most likely to be associated.

(A) Patent ductus arteriosus
(B) Aortic coarctation
(C) Peripheral pulmonary stenosis
(D) Venous hum
(E) Tetralogy of Fallot

174. An eight-year-old boy is seen for the first time for a routine examination. In the history the mother reports he has recently complained of throbbing headaches. He is in the 10th percentile for weight and the 75th for height. On examination he has injected conjunctivae and deep red-blue nasal mucosa. He has loud aortic and pulmonic valve closure sounds. Bilaterally over the back he has grade II-III/VI harsh continuous murmurs that are also heard in the axillae. Arm blood pressure is 110/70, leg pressure 108/70. His electrocardiogram shows borderline tall R waves for his age in VI.

175. A newborn premature infant is found to have a continuous grade II/VI low pitched harsh murmur in the aortic and pulmonic areas over the back and in the axillae. Pulses are normal, Blood pressure is 60/30 in the left arm. Electrocardiogram is normal. The x-ray shows top normal pulmonary arterial markings. A doppler study fails to show turbulence in the main pulmonary artery.

176. A four-year-old girl is brought to the emergency room because of dizziness while playing in the sun. She is accompanied by an adult baby-sitter who is not aware of her medical history other than that she had an emergency operation shortly after birth for blueness. She has a left lateral chest incision. There is a grade III/VI low pitched harsh ejection systolic murmur over her left back. Blood pressure in her arms and legs are equal, 105/30. On x-ray there is evidence of notching of upper left ribs.

Questions 177–180

For each syndrome listed below, select the major cardiovascular abnormality with which it is most likely to be associated.

(A) Atrial septal defect
(B) Ventricular septal defect
(C) Patent ductus arteriosus
(D) Supravalvular aortic stenosis
(E) Peripheral pulmonic stenosis

177. Ellis-van Creveld syndrome

178. Trisomy 18

179. Holt-Oram syndrome

180. Cri-du-chat syndrome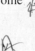

The Cardiovascular System

Answers

126. The answer is C. *(Braunwald, ed 2. p 954. Nadas, ed 3. pp 271–272.)* The major clinical manifestation of digitalis toxicity in infants is vomiting. Affected infants also exhibit certain electrocardiographic changes, including sinus arrhythmia and a wandering pacemaker, paroxysmal tachycardia, and a heart rate of less than 100 beats per minute. Digitalis intoxication appears to be increasing dramatically in frequency, in part because of the widespread use of more potent preparations of the drug. The commonly used digitalis preparation in infants is digoxin. Digoxin blood levels of 2 ng/100 ml or less are usually therapeutic in adults; in contrast, therapeutic digoxin blood levels in infants range from 1 to 5 ng/100 ml.

127. The answer is C. *(Nadas, ed 3. p 295. Watson, pp 690–691.)* Short stature, neck webbing, sexual infantilism, hyperextensible elbows, and a shieldlike chest with widely spaced nipples are signs of Turner's syndrome, which is associated with an XO genotype. Aortic coarctation and pulmonic stenosis are the cardiovascular defects that occur most frequently in individuals who have this disorder. Down's syndrome most commonly is associated with atrial septal defects and endocardial cushion defects; Marfan's syndrome with dilatation of the pulmonary artery and mitral and aortic regurgitation; and Ellis-van Creveld syndrome with an atrial septal defect or single atrium.

128. The answer is B. *(Nadas, ed 3. p 26.)* Infants who have transposition of the great vessels classically present with cyanosis during the first few days after birth. Pulmonary vasculature is engorged. The cardiac contour in infants who have transposition often is described as an "egg on a string." The egg-shaped contour is a result of general enlargement of the heart (due to increased cardiac volume) accompanied by a narrowing of the left upper cardiac border because of the "missing" pulmonary artery at that site. The "string" is the narrow superior mediastinal shadow produced by the anteroposterior alignment of the aorta and main pulmonary artery. Cineangiocardiography can establish with certainty the presence of transposition.

129. The answer is D. *(Roberts, p 390. Keith, ed 3. p 4157.)* The incidence of congenital heart disease in the population is 1 percent. The risk of congenital heart disease in a family with one child born with heart disease is 1 to 4 percent. If there are two children with congenital heart disease the risk escalates to 3 to 12 percent. Mothers with congenital heart disease have offspring with a 14 percent incidence of congenital heart disease. As a subgroup children of mothers with congenital ventricular outflow obstruction have a 23 percent incidence of congenital heart defects.

130. The answer is A. *(Keith, ed 3. p 28.)* The harsh pansystolic murmur heard best in the third and fourth left intercostal spaces along the left sternal border and radiating to the apex is the classical murmur of a ventricular septal defect. An atrial septal defect would not cause a pansystolic murmur. Aortic and pulmonic regurgitation both cause diastolic murmurs, but neither has a rumbling quality. The aortic regurgitant flow may cause mitral vibrations heard at the apex. The quality is higher pitched and more likely blowing or harsh. Also these diastolic murmurs are heard in the pulmonic and aortic areas and may radiate down the sternal borders and in the case of aortic stenosis may be heard to the apex. A rumbling murmur that is very low-pitched is usually generated across an atrioventricular valve. With both atrial and ventricular septal defects if the flow across the defect is large there may be a sufficiently large flow across the tricuspid valve (ASD) or mitral valve (VSD) to generate a diastolic rumbling murmur due to relative atrioventricular valve stenosis. Because the baby has a pansystolic murmur and develops the rumbling apical murmur, he likely has progressively increasing flow from left to right across the ventricular septal defect.

131. The answer is D. *(Schaffer, ed 4. p 240.)* The majority of infants who have aortic atresia cannot be helped by surgery and at best get only temporary relief from medical therapy. These children usually do not survive to one week of age (the average age attained by one series of affected infants was 4.5 days). The prognosis for infants having hypoplasia of the aortic arch may be somewhat better.

132. The answer is A. *(Adams, ed 3. p 14.)* Although pulmonary arterioles are affected by pH and P_{CO_2} as well as by the presence of vasoactive substances, P_{O_2} is considered to be the major regulating influence in the pulmonary arteriolar resistance. The major smooth muscle relaxing effect of a high P_{O_2} causes pulmonary vascular resistance to fall. The theory that tortuosity of the pulmonary vasculature causes elevation of pulmonary vascular resistance is now discounted.

133. The answer is B. *(Nadas, ed 3. pp 462–463.)* Variation in the strength of femoral pulses indicates pressure alterations in the descending aorta, most likely due to a variation in blood flow. In preductal aortic coarctation, blood flow in the descending aorta is affected by a patent ductus arteriosus, which may close intermittently or even permanently. This effect would not occur in a postductal aortic coarctation with a patent ductus arteriosus, because the descending aortic flow is by way of collateral vessels. Due to aortic runoff, pulses in children who have a ventricular septal defect with a patent ductus would be consistently full. The closing of a patent ductus in children with tetralogy of Fallot likely would result in marked cyanosis. Children with preductal aortic coarctation may obtain temporary relief in the situation described in the question by infusion of E-type prostaglandin.

134. The answer is C. *(Nadas, ed 3. p 287.)* Tall stature, long digits, and progressive scoliosis point to a diagnosis of Marfan's disease, an inherited disorder of collagen metabolism. Affected children frequently suffer from mitral regurgitation caused by papillary muscle dysfunction; aortic regurgitation due to dilatation of the valve rings also is common. Pulmonic regurgitation stemming from pulmonary artery dilatation, though it too can occur, is much less common in children who have Marfan's disease than are disturbances of the aortic or mitral valves.

135. The answer is C. *(Nadas, ed 3. p 221.)* The clinical picture presented in the question suggests the presence of an aberrant left coronary artery arising from the pulmonary artery. Electrocardiograms of these infants, in addition to showing nonspecific ST-T changes, often reveal deep Q waves in leads I and aVL and QR or Q-S complexes in V_2, V_3, and V_4. These electrocardiographic changes indicate the presence of infarction and can confirm a diagnosis of an aberrant left coronary artery suggested by clinical examination.

136. The answer is E. *(Friedman, pp 192–193, 207. Nadas, ed 3. pp 228–233.)* Endocardial fibroelastosis is a primary myocardial disease that is characterized by hyperplasia of the elastic tissue of the endocardium. Symptoms, which typically include those of congestive heart failure, usually manifest suddenly in children between the ages of four and ten months. In contrast, an aberrant left coronary artery produces symptoms in neonates. Myocarditis does not produce electrocardiographic evidence of hypertrophy; and Pompe's disease characteristically includes large tongue and hypotonia. Heart failure in infancy rarely is due to idiopathic hypertropic subaortic stenosis.

137. The answer is C. *(Braunwald, ed 2. p 1053.)* All of these conditions can be associated with prolonged fever and a limp due to arthralgia as well as exanthem, adenopathy, and pharyngitis. Conjunctivitis, however, is most likely in Kawasaki disease. The fissured lips, while common in Kawasaki disease, could occur after a long period of fever from any cause if the child became dehydrated. The predominance of neutrophils and high sedimentation rate are common to all. An increase in platelets, however, is found only in Kawasaki disease. Kawasaki disease presents a picture of prolonged fever, rash, epidermal peeling on the hands and feet, especially around the fingertips, ocular conjunctivitis, lymphadenopathy, fissured lips, oropharyngeal mucosal erythema, and arthralgia or arthritis. The diagnosis is still possible in the absence of one or two of these physical findings. The cardiovascular abnormality, if present, involves aneurysms of systemic arteries, especially the coronary arteries.

138. The answer is A. *(Keith, ed 3. p 928–933.)* The presence of pallor, dyspnea, tachypnea, tachycardia, and cardiomegaly are findings that are commonly found in congestive heart failure regardless of the cause. The lack of echocardiographic findings other than ventricular and left atrial dilation and poor ventricular function is inconsistent with both glycogen storage disease of the heart, in which there is muscle thickening, and pericarditis, since there is no pericardial effusion. It is also not consistant with an aberrant origin of the left coronary artery although the origin of the coronary arteries may be more easily missed. On electrocardiogram, the voltages of the ventricular complexes seen with aberrant origin of the left coronary artery are not diminished. Those from the left ventricle are usually high in endocardial fibroelastosis and both right and left ventricular forces are high in glycogen storage disease of the heart.

139. The answer is C. *(Schaffer, ed 4. p 260.)* The presence of a pansystolic murmur in the infant described in the question makes a diagnosis of anomalous pulmonary venous return unlikely. A ventricular septal defect that is either an isolated lesion or associated with other defects can cause a pansystolic murmur; isolated ventricular septal defects rarely cause cyanosis. Although truncus arteriosus occasionally causes a pansystolic murmur, it usually causes a continuous murmur. The presence of a right aortic arch is found in 25 percent of children who have tetralogy of Fallot and therefore increases the likelihood of this diagnosis in the situation presented. As the child becomes older, the degree of right ventricular outflow obstruction is likely to increase, causing persistent cyanosis and a change in the murmur to systolic ejection.

140. The answer is E. *(Braunwald, ed 2. p 946.)* In a fetus, aortic and pulmonary arterial pressures are equal because of the large size of the ductus arteriosus. As a result of the equalization of pressures, blood flow to the fetal organs is determined primarily by local vascular resistance. This resistance may, in turn, be affected by pH, P_{CO_2}, P_{O_2}, or circulating vasoactive agents.

141. The answer is B. *(Schaffer, ed 4. pp 134, 249–250, 267.)* Infants born with the infracardiac variety of total anomalous pulmonary venous return have obstruction to the drainage of pulmonary veins. This anomaly results in a marked degree of pulmonary vascular congestion. Despite the presence of heart failure, cardiomegaly does not develop because of the decreased venous return to the heart. Transposition of the great vessels and pulmonic atresia usually produce cardiomegaly; and mitral stenosis can be expected to be accompanied by evidence of a large left atrium. Hyaline membrane disease in a term infant is unlikely.

142. The answer is C. *(Braunwald, ed 2. p 1686.)* Hypoxic stimulation of the kidneys is thought to cause the release of erythropoietin that stimulates production of red blood cells in the bone marrow. A substrate manufactured in the liver is converted into erythropoietin, most likely in a reaction catalyzed by erythrigenin, an enzyme produced in the kidneys. Aside from inducing production of red blood cells, erythropoietin also increases the rate of erythrocyte production and causes the release of immature reticulocytes into the blood.

143. The answer is E. *(Adams, ed 3. p 733. Behrman, ed 12. pp 1171–1172.)* Congestive heart failure from any cause can result in mild cyanosis, even in the absence of a right-to-left shunt, and poor peripheral pulses when cardiac output is low. Congestive heart failure usually is associated with a rapid pulse rate (up to 200 beats per minute). A pulse rate greater than 200 beats per minute, however, should suggest the presence of a tachyarrhythmia.

144. The answer is A. *(Braunwald, ed 2. p 1626.)* Syncopal episodes in children are not common. Evaluation of children presenting with syncope should include electrocardiography, because a prolonged Q-T interval can be associated with syncope. It is less likely that syncopy in a three-year-old child would be caused by asymmetric septal hypertrophy; echocardiography is the procedure best able to evaluate this disorder.

145. The answer is D. *(Braunwald, ed 2. p 942.)* Ventricular septal defect is by far the most common congenital cardiac defect, constituting about 30 percent of all congenital cardiac anomalies. Atrial septal defect and patent ductus arteriosus each account for about 10 percent of congenital heart abnormalities, and pulmonic stenosis 7 percent. Tetralogy of Fallot, the most common cyanotic lesion, has a 6 percent incidence among neonates with congenital cardiac defects.

146. The answer is D. *(Perloff, ed 2. pp 93–96, 119, 137.)* A loud systolic ejection murmur in the aortic area occurs with valvular, discrete subvalvular, and supravalvular aortic stenosis, but only supravalvular aortic stenosis is associated with development abnormalities. These patients are described as having elfin faces and very often suffer some degree of mental retardation. A bicuspid valve will more likely be associated with regurgitation and, therefore, a diastolic murmur. A brisk right brachial and weaker left brachial pulse are frequent findings in supravalvular aortic stenosis and are thought to be due to the jet of blood directed into the innominate artery by the supravalvular narrowing, causing the more prominent pulse on the right. For the same reason, the right arm blood pressure is about 10 to 15 mm higher than the left. With coarctation of the aorta, the left arm blood pressure and pulse may be less than in the right arm if the left subclavian artery is narrowed by the coarcted portion of the aorta. However, in aortic coarctation one would expect higher pressure in the right arm than in the leg.

147. The answer is A. *(Nadas, ed 3. p 262.)* The greatest cause of congestive heart failure in children is congenital heart disease. Congestive heart failure due to congenital heart disease most often occurs in infants during their first weeks of life. Other etiologies of heart failure in young infants include primary myocardial disease and paroxysmal atrial tachycardia; other causes, such as bacterial endocarditis and rheumatic heart disease, are rare in the first year of life.

148. The answer is C. *(Nadas, ed 3. pp 322–333.)* Children who have an atrial septal defect also may have right ventricular hypertrophy. A loud pulmonic component of the second sound occurs with development of pulmonary arterial hypertension. This is usually of the reversible variety during childhood.

149. The answer is D. *(Nadas, ed 3. pp 598–600.)* A quadruple rhythm associated with the murmur of tricuspid regurgitation and pulmonic stenosis is sufficient to make the diagnosis of Ebstein's anomaly (downward displacement of the tricuspid valve). The presence of P pulmonale (tall P waves in leads II and III) and right ventricular conduction defects confirms the diagnosis. Both tricuspid regurgitation with pulmonic stenosis and tetralogy of Fallot give electrocardiographic evidence of right ventricular enlargement. The Wolff-Parkinson-White syndrome, which frequently accompanies Ebstein's malformation, is not associated with murmurs or cyanosis as an isolated entity.

150. The answer is B. *(Nadas, ed 3. pp 338–339.)* Maldevelopment resulting in ostium primum atrial septal defects also causes displacement of the atrioventricular node. As a result, leftward deviation of the electrocardiographic axis is seen. First-degree atrioventricular block occurs in some patients who have primum atrial defects. Incomplete right bundle-branch block very commonly accompanies secundum atrial septal defects.

151. The answer is B. *(Keith, ed 3. pp 279, 286–288.)* The child described in the question, who has no cyanosis or murmur, no cardiac or pulmonary vascular abnormalities by chest x-ray, and no evidence of structural anomalies by echocardiogram, is unlikely to have an underlying gross anatomic defect. The electrocardiographic pattern in figure B shows the configuration of preexcitation, the pattern seen in the Wolff-Parkinson-White syndrome (WPW). These patients have an aberrant atrioventricular conduction pathway which causes the early ventricular depolarization appearing on the electrocardiograms as a shortened PR interval. The initial slow ventricular depolarization wave is referred to as the delta wave. Seventy percent of patients with WPW have single or repeated episodes of paroxysmal supraventricular tachycardia, which can cause the symptoms described in the question. The preexcitation electrocardiographic pattern and WPW can occur in Ebstein's malformation, but this is unlikely in the absence of cyanosis and with a normal echocardiogram. Ventricular tachycardia is unlikely with WPW. If this were present, the symptoms are likely to be more profound. Active play in a healthy four-year-old child rarely causes symptoms such as those described in the question, but in children with WPW it can occasionally precipitate paroxysmal supraventricular tachycardia.

152. The answer is B. *(Schaffer, ed 4. pp 226, 288.)* During the first day of life, an infant's pulse rate can range from 70 to 180 beats per minute (average: 125); during the first week, the rate varies between 100 and 190 beats per minute (average: 140). A heart rate that persistently falls below 70 beats per minute almost invariably indicates congenital atrioventricular block, which is of the complete type in nearly all cases. Affected infants often present only with bradycardia; however, cyanosis, cardiomegaly, and heart failure can ensue, especially if the pulse rate falls below 50 beats per minute; these children would require cardiac pacing.

153. The answer is B. *(Nadas, ed 3. pp 148–149.)* Rheumatoid arthritis frequently causes spindle-shaped swelling of finger joints and may involve unusual joints such as the sternoclavicular joint. This disorder can be associated with spiking high fevers, which are not a feature of rheumatic fever, toxic synovitis, septic arthritis, or osteoarthritis. Although septic arthritis may affect any joint, it would not be likely to affect finger joints by causing spindle-shaped swellings; in this respect, septic arthritis resembles acute rheumatic fever. Toxic synovitis usually involves hip joints in boys, and osteoarthritis is not a disease of childhood.

154. The answer is B. *(Keith, ed 3. pp 487, 568.)* Transposition of the great vessels with an intact ventricular septum presents with early cyanosis, a normal-sized heart, normal or slightly increased pulmonary vascular markings, and an electrocardiogram showing right axis deviation and right ventricular hypertrophy. In asymptomatic tetralogy of Fallot, cyanosis is unlikely in the first few days of life. Tricuspid atresia, a cause of early cyanosis, causes diminished pulmonary arterial blood flow; the pulmonary fields on x-ray demonstrate a diminution of pulmonary vascularity. There is a left axis and left ventricular hypertrophy by electrocardiogram. Total anomalous pulmonary venous return below the diaphragm is associated with obstruction to pulmonary venous return and a classical radiographic finding of marked fluffy-appearing pulmonary venous congestion. In pulmonic atresia with intact ventricular septum, cyanosis appears early, the lung markings are normal to diminished, and the heart is large.

155. The answer is C. *(Nadas, ed 3. p 295.)* Among the wide variety of cardiac defects associated with Down's syndrome, the most common are endocardial cushion defects and atrial septal defects (ostium secundum). Evidence indicates that half of all children affected by trisomy 21 have congenital heart disease; estimates of the percent of Down's syndrome children who have cardiac anomalies range from a low of 7 percent to a high of 70 percent. Some cardiac lesions, such as tetralogy of Fallot and coarctation of the aorta, have been found to occur with less frequency in children who have Down's syndrome than in controls; other anomalies, like transposition of the great vessels, do not seem to be associated at all with the disorder.

156. The answer is D. *(Nadas, ed 3. pp 322–323, 531, 535, 537.)* Valvular pulmonic stenosis, atrial septal defect, partial anomalous pulmonary venous return, and supravalvular pulmonic stenosis all are associated with a pulmonic ejection murmur. The latter three disorders can result in an increase in pulmonary pressure distal to the pulmonic valve and, as a consequence, accentuation of the pulmonic valve closure sound (as in the patient described in the question); valvular pulmonic stenosis, however, causes diminution of the pulmonic closure sound. The pulmonary artery segment may be enlarged in all four disorders, either from increased flow or due to poststenotic eddy currents that dilate the vessel. Peripheral pulmonary arterial markings usually will be normal or slightly decreased in stenotic lesions but increased in the presence of atrial septal defects (due to elevated pulmonary flow) and partial anomalous pulmonic venous return that is sufficient to cause right ventricular hypertrophy. Thus, the presence of normal pulmonary vascular markings in the child described, in conjunction with the other physical findings, points to a diagnosis of supravalvular pulmonic stenosis.

157. The answer is B (1, 3). *(Braunwald, ed 2. p 948.)* Infants who are in congestive heart failure usually are hyperpneic, if they have hypoxemia and acidemia, or tachypneic, if they have volume overload of the pulmonary circuit. Grunting is associated primarily with pulmonary disease, and periodic breathing with disease of the central nervous system.

158. The answer is D (4). *(Braunwald, ed 2. pp 1684–1685. Roberts, p. 246–247.)* In primary polycythemia there is an increased hematocrit, increased blood volume, and increased cardiac output. In secondary polycythemia there is a decrease in flow with increasing hematocrit. Neither of these mechanisms is responsible for the normal rise in blood pressure seen as children advance in age. Hyperkinetic circulating states are usually associated with high cardiac output. A study of subjects whose age ranged from 15 to 19 years demonstrated that the theory that blood pressure elevation in this age group is related to increased cardiac activity and ouput cannot be supported. The conclusion was that the gradual increase in blood pressure with age is a function of a progressive increase in peripheral vascular resistance from early in life.

159. The answer is A (1, 2, 3). *(Schaffer, ed 4. pp 238–239, 290–291.)* Reduced blood flow through the left ventricle results in underdevelopment of this chamber of the heart. Aortic atresia, mitral atresia, and hypoplasia of the aortic arch, either individually or in combination, can cause this reduction in flow and lead to endocardial fibroelastosis. Isolated endocardial fibroelastosis, however, is not associated with development of a small left ventricle.

160. The answer is A (1, 2, 3). *(Adams, ed 3. pp 268–269.)* Pulmonic stenosis usually is associated with a small-chambered right ventricle that, even following valvotomy, will not allow adequate blood flow into the pulmonary artery. Affected infants require maintenance of their aorticopulmonary shunts. Surgical aorticopulmonary anastomosis, when possible, is the best treatment; infiltration of the ductus arteriosus with formalin has been used for patients who, for anatomical reasons, cannot undergo anastomosis. Prostaglandin (type E) infusion, a temporary emergency measure, can maintain ductal patency until surgery is performed.

161. The answer is A (1, 2, 3). *(Braunwald, ed 2. pp 824–825.)* The major factor in rapid fall of the pulmonary arterial resistance is pulmonary arterial vasodilation resulting from the increased P_{O_2}, to which vessels are exposed. Inflation of the lungs allows the vessels to expand, which is the initial cause of reduction of the resistance. Ductus arteriosus closure, which is brought about by the increase in P_{O_2} plus the change in local prostaglandin, results in a fall in pulmonary arterial pressure. The pressure, if high, retards vasodilation. The enhanced volume due to foramen ovale closure is noncontributory.

162. The answer is A (1, 2, 3). *(Behrman, ed 12. pp 396–397.)* Infants born to diabetic mothers commonly have hypoglycemia, hypocalcemia, and hyperinsulinemia; hyperbilirubinemia also is more common in these infants than in infants of nondiabetic mothers. Newborn infants who are severely hypoglycemic may develop profound congestive heart failure. Even without associated cardiac lesions, murmurs of tricuspid insufficiency may appear due to marked cardiac dilation and persistent fetal pulmonary circulation.

163. The answer is A (1, 2, 3). *(Braunwald, ed 2. pp 1654–1655. Nadas, ed 3. pp 147, 152–155.)* Administration of salicylates and steroids can relieve the inflammatory manifestations of acute rheumatic fever. Salicylates alone usually are sufficient to treat affected children who do not have severe carditis. Neither salicylates nor corticosteroids have an effect on chorea, which is a noninflammatory process.

164. The answer is B (1, 3). *(Keith, ed 3. pp 269, 279–280, 292, 700–701.)* In a child presenting with a seizure, cardiac causes, even though less likely than neurologic causes, must be considered. Ventricular arrhythmia may cause syncope resembling a seizure. Long Q-T syndrome, aortic stenosis, and primary hypertension can all cause ventricular fibrillation with stress. Atrial tachycardia may cause heart failure but does not cause syncope. If aortic stenosis were present, there would be a loud systolic ejection murmur with a thrill. The hearing deficit suggests the possibility of the Jervell-Lange-Nielsen syndrome, the recessive form of the long Q-T syndrome, which is associated with congenital hearing deficit. The mildly accentuated second sound is difficult to evaluate in a child with a thin chest wall, as is the recent onset of fatigue. These two findings, however, may be seen in pulmonary hypertension.

165. The answer is A (1, 2, 3). *(Nadas, ed 3. pp 406–407, 413–414, 417–418.)* The continuous flow of blood through a truncus arteriosus into the pulmonary vessel gives rise to a continuous murmur. Similarly, the continuous blood flow through bronchial collateral vessels can cause a continuous murmur in children who have tetralogy of Fallot. In total anomalous pulmonary venous return, the flow through the pulmonary venous trunk carrying the blood from the pulmonary veins to the right heart may result in a continuous murmur. The murmur associated with patent ductus arteriosus is continuous and affected only to a minor degree by position or respiration, but patients are not cyanotic; in patent ductus arteriosus complicated by pulmonary hypertension, flow through the ductus is not continuous and, therefore, neither is the murmur.

166. The answer is A (1, 2, 3). *(Schaffer, ed 4. pp 247–248.)* A large number of newborn infants who have preductal aortic coarctation are symptomatic within a week or two after birth. Development of heart failure is especially likely if this lesion, or postductal aortic coarctation, is associated with a large left-to-right shunt at the ventricular level. Although patent ductus arteriosus alone may cause early failure in the newborn period, the combination of a ductus with a ventricular septal defect is very likely to result in failure due to marked left ventricular volume overload resulting from the combined shunt. Infants who have tetralogy of Fallot have large ventricular septal defects as part of that lesion; they do not, however, have large left-to-right shunts, because right ventricular pressure is elevated due to the pulmonic and subpulmonic stenosis associated with tetralogy of Fallot.

167. The answer is D (4). *(Nadas, ed 3. pp 335, 598, 631–633.)* Atrioventricularis communis, an ostium primum defect, Ebstein's anomaly, and corrected transposition of the great vessels all may be associated with atrioventricular conduction delay. Tachyarrhythmia is associated frequently with Ebstein's malformation and corrected transposition of the great vessels; and a QR pattern may be present in V_1 in either of these conditions. In Ebstein's malformation, however, a right bundle-branch block pattern is frequently present, and the appearance of a pansystolic murmur is unusual. Although a pansystolic murmur also may be present in children who have atrioventricularis communis, these children are in considerable distress before the age of three years. A pansystolic murmur would not be present in children who have an isolated ostium primum atrial septal defect. Thus, the only condition of those listed in the question that would be likely to be compatible with the clinical picture presented is corrected transposition, which is associated with mitral regurgitation and a ventricular septal defect.

168. The answer is C (2, 4). *(Anderson, vol. 5. p 385.)* For mitral regurgitation medical management alone is not likely to provide the necessary level of cardiac compensation even with the addition of a vasodilator (to reduce afterload) to the usual therapy of digoxin and diuretics needed to improve contractibility and to reduce preload. The child will require closure of any significant left-to-right shunts and, at the least, considerable reduction of mitral regurgitation. Although the obliteration of even complex shunts is usually not a problem for experienced surgeons, surgery involving the mitral valve may be extremely difficult because of grossly abnormal leaflets and suspensory structures. Replacement of the valve with a bioprosthetic homograft valve or a prosthetic valve may be possible in the larger infant, but the replacement may be too large for the small infant's valve ring. The prosthetic valve orifices are too obstructive in the small overall size needed. A homograft valve, although less obstructive, in time undergoes leaflet deterioration. The use of the prosthetic valve requires long-term anticoagulation, a problem in small children. Both types of artificial valves require replacement as the child grows. The better approach is to repair rather than to replace the valve, accepting a mild-to-moderate degree of regurgitation that will be manageable using medical therapy.

169. The answer is E (all). *(Keith, ed 3. p 538.)* In all patients with tricuspid atresia there is need for a nonrestrictive communication across the atrial septum to allow the systemic venous return to the functioning ventricle. In addition these patients may require operative aorticopulmonary shunts to provide blood flow to the lungs. In the rare situations in which there is excessive blood flow into the pulmonary circuit pulmonary banding may be necessary to reduce the excessive pulmonary flow.

170. The answer is B (1, 3). *(Perloff, ed 3. pp 299–302.)* As in atrial septal defects, the increased flow across the pulmonic valve due to the shunt causes a pulmonic flow murmur. The increased right ventricular volume results in a prominent right ventricular impulse (heave). The pulmonic second sound (P_2) is accentuated only in the presence of pulmonary hypertension. Wide and fixed splitting of the second heart sound, which classically occurs with atrial septal defects with significant flows, does not occur with the increased flow into the right atrium secondary to partial anomalous venous return with intact atrial septum. The variation in right ventricular and left ventricular filling that normally occurs with inspiration does not occur with atrial septal defect. In atrial septal defect with inspiration, right ventricular volume increases due to caval return. Shunting decreases due to the increase in pulmonary impedance, resulting in increased left ventricular filling. There is thus a delay of both the aortic component of the second sound and the pulmonic second sound. During expiration, right ventricular volume is again increased, but by increase in shunt. The latter results in a smaller left ventricular volume. The result is splitting during inspiration and expiration.

171. The answer is A (1, 2, 3). *(Roberts, pp 368–369.)* Premature infants with patent ductus arteriosus refractory to medical management had a mortality rate of 11 percent and an incidence of enterocolitis of similar magnitude. With surgical management the mortality rate was 9 percent and the rate of enterocolitis 0.30 percent. The value of surgical patent ductus closure when the infant is refractory to medical management is clear from these findings.

172.   The answer is E (all). *(Perloff, ed 3. pp 344–350.)* The embryonic endocardial cushions are responsible for the conjoining of the lower (primum) portion of
the atrial septum and the upper portion of the ventricular septum, as well as the
development of the anterior mitral leaflet and septal leaflet of the tricuspid valve.
Maldevelopment of the cushions can result, depending on degree, in a single or
combination of defects: ostium primum atrial septal defect, ventricular septal defect, mitral or tricuspid regurgitation, or when severe, complete atrioventricular
canal defect with communication of all four heart chambers.

173.   The answer is A (1, 2, 3). *(Watson, p 514.)* With increased obstruction to
right ventricular outflow, the pulmonic ejection click of valvular pulmonic stenosis becomes quieter and occurs earlier. On the other hand, increased stenosis
causes an increase in the grade of the systolic murmur. Due to prolongation of
right ventricular emptying, pulmonic valve closure is extended beyond aortic
valve closure.

174–176.   The answers are: 174-C, 175-C, 176-E. *(Keith, ed 3. pp 29, 425, 478,
494, 741, 792–793.)* Patent ductus arteriosus presents its classical clinical findings of a continuous harsh murmur over the right upper chest, wide pulse pressure, and bounding pulses when there is a significant left-to-right shunt through it.
Early, unless the flow is torrential, the pulmonary vascular markings may not be
clearly increased. The radiation of the continuous ductal murmur, especially in
small infants, may be throughout the chest, but it tends not to be of bilaterally
equal grade. Flow from left to right occurs once the pulmonary resistance falls
sufficiently below peripheral systemic resistance. The collateral circulation associated with *aortic coarctation* may cause a continuous murmur that is heard in the
interscapular area. Lower extremity pulses and leg pressures are diminished in
relation to those in the upper extremities. Headaches are not usual in aortic coarctation until there is a cerebrovascular accident secondary to the aneurysm
formation which can occur in untreated patients in adolescence or adulthood. In
the patient described the headache is more likely from sinusitis.

   Peripheral pulmonary arterial stenosis usually involves the branches beyond
the right and left primary branches. There are less common variations involving in
addition the main pulmonary artery, its bifurcation bilaterally or rarely unilaterally. The flow as in patent ductus arteriosus is dependent on the fall in the pulmonary arteriolar resistance to a level sufficient to permit the turbulence clinically
appreciated as a murmur. The flow through the arterial narrowing is continuous.

The murmurs can vary from ejection systolic to continuous depending on the pulmonary flow and the degree of narrowing of the stenotic areas. As the narrowings are primarily bilateral, the murmurs are usually heard symetrically over the lungs.

Venous hums are most commonly heard below the clavicles and over the base of the heart. The hums may be bilateral or one-sided. The hums may be altered or obliterated by head turning and extension or by pressure applied over the neck veins. Patients with *tetralogy of Fallot* may have continuous murmurs over the back due to flow through collateral vessels from the aorta to the pulmonary arteries. The murmurs may be symetrical or, on occasion, more one-sided. In those patients with tetralogy of Fallot who have been treated with an aortico-pulmonary surgical shunt there will be a harsh continuous murmur that is heard best on the side of the lung into which the aortic blood enters the pulmonary artery. The Blalock-Taussig surgical shunt (connection of the subclavian artery to the like-sided primary pulmonary arterial branch) may result in rib notching of the uppermost ribs on the side of the surgical anastomosis.

177–180. The answers are: 177-A, 178-B, 179-A, 180-B. *(Braunwald, ed 2. p 943.)* The Ellis-van Creveld syndrome is an autosomal recessive trait. The common cardiac defects occur in 50 to 60 percent of affected individuals, commonly a secundum atrial septal defect. This may be associated with some variant of hypoplastic left heart syndrome. The characteristic skeletal findings are short stature from birth, distal extremity shortening, and bilateral polydactyly. The latter permits an in utero diagnosis.

The common intracardiac defect in children with trisomy 18 is a ventricular septal defect. Patent ductus arteriosus is also commonly present. The cardiac defects are usually major and often result in heart failure, which is a significant factor in the early death of these children.

The Holt-Oram syndrome is one of the rare disorders in which a secundum atrial septal defect seems to be the result of a single dominant gene. Ventricular septal defect is the second most common cardiac anomaly. The most common hand/arm defect is a fingerlike appearance of one or both thumbs. First degree relatives of patients with Holt-Oram syndrome have a 50 percent incidence of atrial septal defects, as opposed to a 3 percent occurrence in the sporadically occurring type of atrial septal defect.

Children with cri-du-chat (literally, cat cry) syndrome have a chromosomal abnormality. The associated cardiac anomaly is a ventricular septal defect. There is microcephaly, an antimongoloid slant of the palperbral fissures, and severe mental retardation.

The Gastrointestinal Tract

John B. Watkins

DIRECTIONS: Each question below contains five suggested answers. Choose the **one best** response to each question.

181. All of the following factors can be associated with an increased risk of neurologic damage in a jaundiced newborn EXCEPT

(A) metabolic acidosis
(B) sulfisoxazole therapy
(C) the presence of reducing substances in the urine
(D) maternal ingestion of aspirin during pregnancy
(E) maternal ingestion of phenobarbital during pregnancy

Questions 182–183

A three-day-old infant is noted in the newborn nursery to be jaundiced. Total serum bilirubin level is 10.5 mg/100 ml (direct, 0.5 mg/100ml).

182. Additional physical findings or historical factors that could be associated with this infant include all of the following EXCEPT

(A) breast-feeding
(B) normal-size liver
(C) history of jaundice in a sibling
(D) family history of Rotor's syndrome
(E) family history of hereditary spherocytosis

183. Which of the following laboratory findings would be consistent with the diagnosis of physiologic jaundice in the infant described above?

(A) An elevated peripheral normoblast cell count
(B) An elevated level of hepatic glucuronyl transferase
(C) An elevated level of serum glutamic-oxaloacetic transaminase
(D) Normal excretion of bromsulphalein
(E) None of the above

184. Which of the following malabsorptive conditions principally influences the intestinal or mucosal phase of digestion?

(A) Zollinger-Ellison syndrome
(B) Enterokinase deficiency
(C) *Giardia lamblia* infestation
(D) Gastrocolic fistula
(E) Biliary atresia

185. All of the following statements concerning the digestion and absorption of medium-chain triglycerides are true EXCEPT that

(A) bile salts are required for their absorption
(B) they are incorporated into chylomicrons only to a minor degree
(C) during transport they are bound to albumin
(D) they are rapidly hydrolyzed by pancreatic lipase
(E) they are metabolized in the liver

186. A biopsy sample from the small intestine of a child is examined by light microscopy; a photomicrograph is shown below. The diagnosis most compatible with the findings depicted is

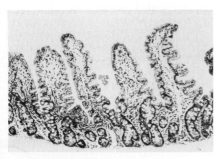

(A) celiac disease
(B) abetalipoproteinemia
(C) Whipple's disease
(D) congenital agammaglobulinemia
(E) sucrase-isomaltase deficiency

187. A child who has primary sucrase-isomaltase deficiency would be likely to have

(A) no family history of the disorder
(B) abnormal small-bowel mucosa
(C) reduced lactase activity
(D) reduced glucose absorption
(E) production of hydrogen following a sucrose load

188. The D-xylose tolerance test may be abnormal in individuals with any of the following conditions that are characterized by malabsorption EXCEPT

(A) celiac disease
(B) pancreatic deficiency
(C) bacterial overgrowth syndrome
(D) short bowel syndrome
(E) regional enteritis

189. Findings that are commonly associated with ulcerative colitis include

(A) rectal bleeding
(B) transmural pathology
(C) perianal abscesses
(D) "skip" lesions
(E) anorectal fistulas

190. Cirrhosis, complicated by portal hypertension, can occur in association with all of the following disorders EXCEPT

(A) cystic fibrosis
(B) alpha$_1$-antitrypsin deficiency
(C) congenital hepatic fibrosis
(D) Wilson's disease
(E) Histocytosis X

191. A three-week-old infant who is still at birthweight has bloody diarrhea. The child had delayed passage of meconium while in the newborn nursery. All of the following disorders should be strongly considered in the differential diagnosis EXCEPT

(A) necrotizing enterocolitis
(B) cystic fibrosis
(C) Hirschsprung's disease
(D) hypothyroidism
(E) salmonellosis

192. A three-year-old girl who has a prominent abdomen and lymphedema of the right arm is admitted to the hospital for investigation of her abdominal distension and persistent diarrhea. Initial laboratory findings include a total serum protein concentration of 3.2 g/100 ml (albumin, 1.2 g/100 ml). Based on these symptoms and laboratory findings, the most likely diagnosis for this child would be

(A) Menetrier's disease
(B) cystic fibrosis
(C) tropical sprue
(D) intestinal lymphangiectasia
(E) severe pulmonic stenosis with heart failure

193. All of the following features would be associated with hepatitis B infection EXCEPT

(A) chronic carrier state
(B) transmission from mother
(C) fulminant hepatitis
(D) live vaccine
(E) glomerulonephritis

194. Which of the following laboratory findings would be consistent with a diagnosis of Reye's syndrome?

(A) Hypoammonemia
(B) Cellular spinal fluid
(C) Leukopenia
(D) Diffusely abnormal electroencephalogram
(E) Shortened prothrombin time

195. A six-week-old dehydrated child is admitted to a hospital following ten days of vomiting. Pyloric stenosis is suspected. Which of the following findings would be most consistent with this diagnosis?

(A) Jaundice and indirect hyperbilirubinemia
(B) Hyponatremia with a hyperchloremic metabolic acidosis
(C) An elevated serum potassium level
(D) A urine specific gravity of 1.005
(E) A urine pH of 4.5

196. In a child who has long-standing cholestasis, the laboratory finding LEAST likely to be exhibited would be

(A) an elevated serum cholesterol level
(B) an elevated serum lipoprotein X level
(C) an elevated vitamin E concentration
(D) an elevated serum alkaline phosphatase level
(E) a normal prothrombin time

197. Which of the following is LEAST associated with *Giardia lamblia* infestation?

(A) Fecal-oral contamination
(B) Chronic carrier state
(C) Trophozoites and cysts in stool
(D) Tissue invasion
(E) Contaminated water as the major source

198. A child who has undergone an ileal resection would be likely to exhibit all of the following findings EXCEPT

(A) iron deficiency anemia
(B) renal oxalate stones
(C) an abnormal Schilling test with intrinsic factor
(D) a positive response to cholestyramine therapy
(E) an increase in glycine-conjugated bile acids

199. Which of the following clinical and pathologic findings is most characteristic of Crohn's disease?

(A) Rectal bleeding
(B) Short stature and delayed puberty
(C) Pericholangitis
(D) Toxic megacolon
(E) Small bowel involvement

Questions 200–202

A 14-month-old infant is admitted to the hospital with a six-month history of irritability, developmental delay, and failure to thrive; malnutrition is suspected.

200. Which of the following growth patterns would be most characteristic of a child with malnutrition?

(A) Subnormal weight, normal height and head circumference
(B) Subnormal weight and height, normal head circumference
(C) Subnormal weight and head circumference, normal height
(D) Subnormal head circumference, normal weight and height
(E) Subnormal weight, height, and head circumference

201. Additional diagnostic tests that should be ordered for the child described include all of the following EXCEPT

(A) 72-hour stool collection for fat
(B) thyroid scan
(C) complete blood cell count
(D) urinalysis
(E) urine culture

202. All of the following findings support a diagnosis of malnutrition in the child described above due to excessive caloric losses from the gastrointestinal tract EXCEPT

(A) a stool fat concentration greater than 10 percent of intake
(B) a sweat chloride concentration of 75 mg/100 ml
(C) increase in serum xylose at one hour of more than 30 mg/100 ml
(D) the presence of iron deficiency anemia
(E) the presence of multisegmented polymorphonuclear leukocytes

DIRECTIONS: Each question below contains four suggested answers of which **one or more** is correct. Choose the answer:

A	if	**1, 2, and 3**	are correct
B	if	**1 and 3**	are correct
C	if	**2 and 4**	are correct
D	if	**4**	is correct
E	if	**1, 2, 3, and 4**	are correct

203. The x-ray shown below can suggest which of the following diagnoses?

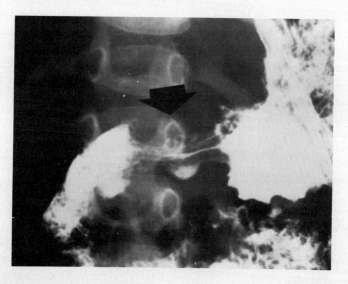

(1) Chronic granulomatous disease
(2) Eosinophilic gastroenteritis
(3) Lymphoma
(4) Crohn's disease

204. The gastrointestinal manifestations of intestinal lymphangectasia include

(1) hypoalbuminema
(2) lymphopenia
(3) chylous ascites
(4) resolution on a low-fat medium-chain triglyceride diet

205. Factors associated with human hepatitis B infection include which of the following?

(1) Oral-fecal exposure and transmission
(2) Dane particles
(3) Migratory arthritis
(4) Surface antigen

206. True statements concerning sulfasalazine (Azulfidine), a commonly used treatment for children who have inflammatory bowel disease, include which of the following?

(1) It contains two pharmacologically active ingredients
(2) It is converted into its active form principally by colonic bacteria
(3) It is excreted after being acetylated in the liver
(4) It is extremely effective in treating children who have Crohn's disease isolated in the small bowel

207. Correct statements concerning Crohn's disease include all of the following EXCEPT that

(1) it typically produces transmural lesions
(2) it can be associated with aphthous stomatitis in children
(3) it is associated with an increased incidence of colonic cancer
(4) it rarely spares the rectum

208. Gastrointestinal manifestations of cystic fibrosis include

(1) portal hypertension and varices
(2) an ileocecal mass
(3) abnormal gallbladder function
(4) constipation and obstruction

209. Which of the following disorders can be associated with disease of the terminal ileum?

(1) Crohn's disease
(2) Schonlein-Henoch purpura
(3) Tuberculosis
(4) *Yersinia enterocolitica* infection

210. Correct statements about achalasia include which of the following?

(1) Lower esophageal sphincter pressure is elevated
(2) Lower esophageal sphincter fails to relax with swallowing
(3) It is associated with vagal and ganglionic degeneration
(4) It is usually associated with pseudoobstruction syndrome

211. Lactose intolerance can be diagnosed by which of the following laboratory studies?

(1) Blood glucose levels before and after oral administration of lactose
(2) Hydrogen excretion in breath after oral administration of lactose
(3) Stool pH and reducing substances
(4) Small intestinal biopsy and enzyme (lactase) assay

212. A six-week-old infant is admitted to a hospital because of jaundice. Which of the following disorders could be responsible for obstructive jaundice in this infant?

(1) Cystic fibrosis
(2) Gilbert's disease
(3) Alpha$_1$-antitrypsin deficiency
(4) Hypothyroidism

213. Which of the following conditions that are characterized by malabsorption are associated with abnormal function of the intestinal mucosa?

(1) Dermatitis herpetiformis
(2) Hartnup disease
(3) Folic acid deficiency
(4) Cystic fibrosis

214. A 30-hour-old male infant, the product of a pregnancy complicated by polyhydramnios, presents with abdominal distension, poor feeding, and recurrent vomiting, the vomitus being bile stained. The infant has passed on meconium-stained stool. There is no evidence of fever, diarrhea, or melena. The physical examination is normal except for abdominal distension, mild jaundice, and hypotonic bowel sounds. A barium enema (see x-ray below) was obtained and reveals a small-diameter colon. A diagnostic and treatment regimen for this infant should consist of

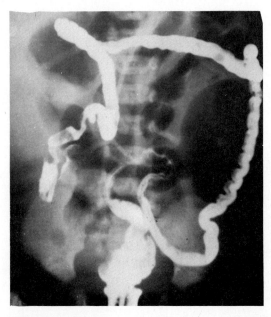

(1) diatrizoate methylglucamine (Gastrografin) enemas
(2) small-bowel surgery
(3) pancreatic enzyme supplements
(4) rectal biopsy for ganglion cells

SUMMARY OF DIRECTIONS

A	B	C	D	E
1,2,3 only	1,3 only	2,4 only	4 only	All are correct

215. An 18-month-old girl was evaluated for poor weight gain and growth during the prior six months, iron deficiency anemia, irritability, decrease in appetite, and diarrhea. An upper gastrointestinal series and small bowel biopsy were performed, the results of which are illustrated below. The possible pathogenic mechanisms operating in this child include which of the following?

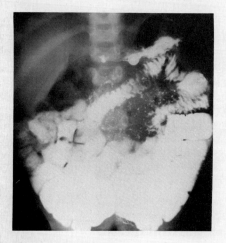
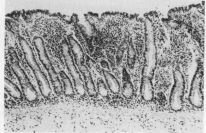

(1) Viral infection
(2) Peptidase deficiency
(3) Endocrine disorder
(4) Immunologic disorder

DIRECTIONS: The groups of questions below consist of lettered choices followed by several numbered items. For each numbered item select the **one** lettered choice with which it is **most** closely associated. Each lettered choice may be used once, more than once, or not at all.

Questions 216–220.

Match the following.

(A) Non-A, non-B hepatitis
(B) Hepatitis B
(C) Both
(D) Neither

216. This is the most common cause of transfusion-related hepatitis

217. Infectious agent is persistent in serum

218. Human disease is transmissible to an animal model

219. Chronic hepatitis occurs commonly

220. Vaccine to prevent the disease is available

Questions 221–225

Match the following.

(A) Wilson's disease
(B) Alpha$_1$-antitrypsin deficiency
(C) Both
(D) Neither

221. Symptoms often appear in the first year of life

222. Inherited as an autosomal recessive trait

223. Can be associated with pulmonary emphysema

224. Causes postnecrotic cirrhosis

235. Can be associated with hemolytic episodes

Questions 226–230

For each description that follows, select the disorder with which it is most likely to be associated.

(A) Peutz-Jeghers syndrome
(B) Gardner's syndrome
(C) Juvenile polyps
(D) Juvenile polyposis of the colon
(E) Lymphoid polyposis

226. Commonly shows malignant degeneration

227. Is associated with soft-tissue masses

228. May be related to *Giardia lamblia* infection

229. Is definitely not inherited

230. Is associated with adenomatous polyps

The Gastrointestinal
Tract

Answers

181. The answer is E. *(Silverman, ed 3. pp 19–21.)* Unconjugated, unbound bilirubin levels above 20 to 25 mg/100 ml in full-term newborn infants can lead to diffusion of bilirubin into brain tissue and thus to neurologic complications. Sulfisoxazole and salicylates compete with bilirubin for binding sites on albumin; therefore, the presence of these drugs can cause serum unbound bilirubin levels to rise. Metabolic acidosis also reduces binding of bilirubin, and the finding of reducing substances in an infant's urine can suggest galactosemia. Administration of phenobarbital has been used to induce glucuronyl transferase in newborn infants and thus can reduce, rather than exacerbate, neonatal jaundice.

182. The answer is D. *(Silverman, ed 3. pp 557–563.)* All of the physical and historical items listed in the question except Rotor's syndrome can be associated with the jaundice of the infant described. A chronic familial disease that is diagnosed only rarely in children, Rotor's syndrome produces elevated levels of serum conjugated bilirubin due to a defect in liver-cell excretion of conjugated bilirubin into the biliary system. It is not a cause of unconjugated hyperbilirubinemia in newborn infants.

183. The answer is E. *(Schaffer, ed 4. pp 641–642.)* The transient elevation of unconjugated bilirubin levels commonly found in newborn infants (physiologic jaundice or hyperbilirubinemia of the newborn) is caused by a temporary deficiency of the hepatic enzyme bilirubin glucuronyl transferase. Aside from an elevation in serum bilirubin levels, infants who have physiologic jaundice typically demonstrate normal laboratory findings. In full-term infants, liver function studies are normal. Defects in coagulation are not observed, and complete blood cell counts are within normal limits. Examination of urine would not show the presence of bile. Tests such as bromsulphalein excretion study, which evaluates conjugation, would be prolonged.

184. The answer is C. *(Silverman, ed 3. pp 262–265.)* The intraluminal phase of digestion involves the hydrolysis and solubilization of fats, proteins, and complex carbohydrates. Acid hypersecretion in individuals who have Zollinger-Ellison syndrome results in the inactivation of pancreatic enzymes and the precipitation of bile salts. Enterokinase deficiency restricts the activation of trypsin. Biliary atresia prevents the excretion of bile salts, and a gastrocolic fistula can lead to bacterial overgrowth of the small intestine. Unlike these disorders, which interfere with the intraluminal phase of digestion, infestation by *Giardia lamblia* causes malabsorption by damaging the intestinal mucosa.

185. The answer is A. *(Greenberger, N Engl J Med 280:1047, 1969.)* Medium-chain triglycerides consist of fatty acids that contain from 8 to 12 carbon atoms. They are rapidly hydrolyzed by pancreatic lipase; and because the fatty acids and monoglycerides are water soluble, bile salts are not necessary for solubilization or absorption. Medium-chain triglycerides, which bypass the usual mucosal pathway of triglyceride resynthesis, are transported (albumin-bound) principally in the portal blood; in the liver they undergo nearly complete metabolism.

186. The answer is E. *(Silverman, ed 3. pp 242–243. Trier, N Engl J Med 285: 1470, 1973.)* When examined by light microscopy, a biopsy sample from the small intestine of an individual who has sucrase-isomaltase deficiency will appear normal. In the other disorders listed in the question, however, histologic examination of the small bowel reveals the presence of diagnostic or at least highly characteristic lesions. In sucrase-isomaltase deficiency, analysis of the intestinal disaccharidase enzymes demonstrate normal lactase activity with an absence of the sucrase enzyme. Therapy should include removal of the offending sugar from the diet.

187. The answer is E. *(Silverman, ed 3. pp 242–243.)* Sucrase-isomaltase deficiency is an inherited autosomal recessive condition characterized by a reduction in or absence of this disaccharidase. As in other disaccharidase deficiencies, such as lactase deficiency, intestinal mucosa is normal on histologic examination of a biopsy sample. Malabsorption of sucrose results in bacterial metabolism of carbohydrate and production of hydrogen. The mechanism of glucose absorption is independent of—and thus unaffected by a deficiency in—sucrase-isomaltase activity.

188. The answer is B. *(Silverman, ed 3. pp 894–895.)* D-Xylose absorption is a measure of mucosal function of the small intestine. Diseases such as gluten-induced enteropathy (celiac disease) and regional enteritis that damage small bowel intestinal mucosa will cause abnormal D-xylose absorption values. Because pancreatic insufficiency disrupts the intraluminal phase of digestion, the mucosal transport is not altered. Patients with short bowel syndrome have decreased absorption due to decreased absorptive surface area.

189. The answer is A. *(Petersdorf, ed 10. pp 1738–1752. Sleisenger, ed 3. pp 1122–1164.)* Ulcerative colitis characteristically is associated with a continuous lesion involving the superficial mucosal tissue of the colon. Rectal bleeding and, especially, bloody diarrhea are major symptoms; however, the severity of the symptoms, the clinical course, and the prognosis are highly variable. Sigmoidoscopic examination typically shows increased mucosal friability and decreased mucosal detail. Anorectal fistulas and perianal abscesses are much more common in individuals who have Crohn's disease. Extraintestinal manifestations, such as skin lesions and liver disease, are not uncommon in association with ulcerative colitis.

190. The answer is C. *(Kerr, Q J Med 30:91–117, 1961. Silverman, ed 3. p 738.)* All of the conditions listed in the question are associated with portal hypertension, and all but congenital hepatic fibrosis are associated with cirrhosis as well. Children who have congenital hepatic fibrosis usually present with portal hypertension and upper gastrointestinal bleeding; their portal hypertension is due to a presinusoidal block, and they have normal liver function. The findings of associated renal lesions and a positive family history help confirm the diagnosis of congenital hepatic fibrosis. In the other disorders listed in the question, liver disease is a primary or associated finding which can be complicated by cirrhosis.

191. The answer is D. *(Schapiro, pp 217–236. Silverman, ed 3. pp 69–70.)* Delayed passage of meconium occurs in a high percentage of children who have Hirschsprung's disease. These children may develop enterocolitic complications, poor weight gain, and diarrhea — rather than constipation — in the first few months of life. Infections including salmonellosis may cause bloody diarrhea in a neonate and occur frequently in association with Hirschsprung's disease. Dilatation, necrosis, perforation, and intramural pneumatosis of the ileum and colon, often with bloody diarrhea, are characteristics of necrotizing enterocolitis, an idiopathic complication of prematurity, exchange transfusions, and severe neonatal infection. Other conditions associated with delayed passage of meconium include a meconium plug, inspissated meconium accompanying cystic fibrosis, and hypothyroidism. An infant who has hypothyroidism, however, usually is constipated; diarrhea rarely occurs in association with this disorder.

192. The answer is D. *(Silverman, ed 3. pp 308–312.)* The child described in the question has abnormally low levels of serum albumin and total serum protein. Intestinal lymphangiectasia is a type of protein-losing enteropathy that probably results from a congenital abnormality of the lymphatic system. It is frequently associated with chronic lymphatic obstruction and lymphedema in various parts of the body, such as the hands, the arms, and especially the legs; this chronic lymphedema is called Milroy's disease. Children who have intestinal lymphangiectasia have hypoproteinemia as a result of protein loss from the small bowel. These children also have lymphocytopenia, which is caused by the loss of lymphocytes by way of the lymph. Other associated findings include abnormal delayed hypersensitivity, hypocalcemia, malabsorption, edema, and occasionally pleural effusions. Treatment with a low-fat diet, supplemented by medium-chain triglycerides, often reduces lymph flow and may be beneficial. Although severe right-sided heart disease and Menetrier's disease both may cause protein loss in the gastrointestinal tract, they rarely are associated with lymphatic aberrations. Diarrhea and growth problems are common to tropical sprue and cystic fibrosis, both of which also can lead to protein loss from the bowel.

193. The answer is D. *(Silverman, ed 3. pp 580–600.)* Hepatitis B infection may result in a chronic carrier state and be transmitted after birth from mother to infant. Fulminant hepatitis and glomerulonephritis secondary to immune complex deposition are recognized complications. Vaccination with good immunity is achieved using a killed inactivated vaccine that does not contain live virus.

194. The answer is D. *(Silverman, ed 3. pp 630–653. Petersdorf, ed 10. pp 1819–1820. Partin, N Engl J Med 285: 1139–1143, 1971. Reye, Lancet 2:749–757, 1963.)* Reye's syndrome is an idiopathic syndrome that usually begins as a mild, nonspecific illness that worsens suddenly, leading to marked abnormalities of the central nervous system, encephalopathy, coma, and hepatic dysfunction. Specific biochemical deficiencies, including deficiency of ornithine transcarbamylase, have been suggested. The urea cycle does not seem to be primarily involved. Serum levels of ammonia, amino acids, and glutamic-oxaloacetic transaminase are elevated in affected children; white blood cell count also is higher than normal. Other laboratory findings include hypoglycemia, prolonged prothrombin time, and acellular cerebrospinal fluid. Mitochondrial lesions predominate in the brain and liver; and, in the proper clinical setting, microvesicular hepatic steatosis is diagnostic for the disorder. Electroencephalographic examination is diffusely abnormal and typically demonstrates high-voltage, slow-wave activity.

195. The answer is A. *(Scharli, J Pediatr Surg 4:108–114, 1969.)* Symptoms of children who have pyloric stenosis include vomiting, dehydration, constipation, moderate jaundice (indirect hyperbilirubinemia), and a palpable mass in the right upper quadrant. The differential diagnosis, particularly in male infants, should include salt loss due to one type of the adrenogenital syndrome; infants with this disorder characteristically are acidotic and have an elevated serum potassium level. In contrast, infants who have pyloric stenosis have metabolic alkalosis and an alkaline, concentrated urine.

196. The answer is C. *(Guggenheim, J Pediatr 100:51–58, 1982.)* Absorption of vitamine E, a lipovitamin, is decreased in children with long-standing cholestasis. The deficiency state is occasionally associated with a sensory neuropathy, optic degeneration, and deficiency of upward gaze. Vitamin E levels must be correlated with total serum lipids when evaluating the deficiency state. Obstructive liver disease causes elevation of serum cholesterol and alkaline phosphatase levels; the serum level of lipoprotein X, an abnormal lipoprotein that accumulates in the absence of proper amounts of lecithin-cholesterol acyltransferase, also is increased. Lipoprotein X is characteristic of cholestatic syndromes. Although prothrombin time is vitamin K-sensitive, it often remains normal until deficiency of this lipid-soluble vitamin becomes severe.

197. The answer is D. *(Sleisenger, ed 3. pp 986–989.)* *Giardia lambia,* the first protozoan parasite to be described, is a common parasitic infestation. It is acquired by ingestion of cysts acquired from contaminated drinking water, with known reservoir hosts being dogs and beavers. Fecal-oral contamination is reported to occur among children. Mechanisms for pathogenesis are not certain, although epithelial damage and secondary dissacharide deficiencies have been documented. Clinical features include prolonged diarrhea and signs of malabsorption such as flatulence, weight loss, and failure to thrive. A chronic carrier state occurs, often in patients with immunodeficiency or hypogammaglobulinemia. Tissue invasion is uncommon. Treatment agents include quinacrine, metronidazole, and tinidazole.

198. The answer is A. *(Petersdorf, ed 10. pp 1720–1730. Sleisenger, ed 3. p 292.)* Functions of the ileum include vitamin B_{12} absorption and absorption of bile salts by an active transport mechanism to complete the enterohepatic circulation of bile salts. Loss of ileal absorption of vitamin B_{12} can lead to the development of pernicious anemia. Excessive loss of bile salts, which can occur in association with ileal resection, may cause diarrhea, which is responsive to cholestyramine therapy, and an increase in glycine-conjugated bile acids. Malabsorption of fat and calcium secondary to bile-salt deficiency may result in increased oxalate absorption and the formation of calcium oxalate renal stones.

199. The answer is E. *(Schiff, ed 4. pp 1373–1378. Silverman, ed 3. pp 337–389. Sleisenger, ed 3. pp 1088–1118.)* Small bowel involvement differentiates ulcerative colitis from Crohn's disease: in the latter any area of the small intestinal tract and colon may be affected, whereas in ulcerative colitis only the colon is involved. Growth failure and delayed puberty may occur in both conditions but are more common in Crohn's disease, often presenting in an insidious fashion. Rectal friability and bleeding are commonly associated with both ulcerative colitis and Crohn's disease, whereas toxic megacolon and pericholangitis are more often complications of ulcerative colitis. Isolated small bowel disease should be differentiated from lymphoma or infection by the appropriate diagnostic procedures before assuming Crohn's disease as the etiology.

200. The answer is A. *(Silverman, ed 3. pp 4–5.)* Most children who are failing to thrive due to malnutrition have a normal head circumference, normal or near-normal height, but a weight that is less than expected given the height. Common causes of malnutrition include inadequate caloric intake, excessive gastrointestinal losses, peripheral disease impairing caloric metabolism, or a combination of these and other causes. Social and cultural factors often are implicated to some extent in the development of malnutrition.

201. The answer is B. *(Silverman, ed 3. pp 7–8.)* In the workup of a child suspected of having malnutrition, a complete nutritional history should be elicited. Furthermore a complete blood cell count, urinalysis, urine culture, and examination for fat in a 72-hour stool sample are essential tests in evaluating nutritional function. Children whose failure to thrive can be traced to thyroid dysfunction or an endocrine disorder would have a different growth pattern (i.e., subnormal weight and height for their age) than the child described in the question.

202. The answer is C. *(Silverman, ed 3. pp 249–261.)* D-Xylose is a poorly absorbed sugar that is not metabolized in the body and thus is excreted intact in the urine. Measurement of xylose concentration in a five-hour urine sample or measurement of blood levels at 0, 30, 60, and 90 minutes provides a good indication of the integrity of the mucosa of the small intestine. For a 14-month-old child, a D-xylose excretion greater than 20 percent or a rise in serum levels of 30 mg/100 ml (dose 0.5 g/kg body weight or 14.5 g/m^2) indicates good mucosal function. A sweat chloride level of 75 mg/100 ml indicates cystic fibrosis; iron deficiency anemia and a stool fat concentration exceeding 10 percent of intake indicate malabsorption; and the presence of multisegmented polymorphonuclear leukocytes indicates a deficiency of folic acid or vitamin B_{12} absorption, either primary or secondary to mucosal dysfunction.

203. The answer is E (all). *(Greseon, Pediatrics 54:456, 1974. Sleisenger, ed 3. pp 162–185.)* The x-ray presented in the question shows antral narrowing, an unusual finding in children. This finding should not be considered as indicating only an ulcer, as it can be associated with all of the disorders listed in the question. Hence, the confirmed diagnosis of these conditions cannot be made on the basis of x-ray alone. A per oral gastric biopsy is necessary in order to differentiate one from the other.

204. Answer is E (all). *(Sleisenger, ed. 3. pp 285–286. Gryboski, ed 2. pp 469–472.)* Intestinal lymphangectasia, presumed to be congenital, is associated with excessive gastrointestinal protein loss and dilatation of the submucosal lymphatics of the small intestine. Lymphopenia is the result of lymphocyte loss from the lymphatics, occasionally to the extent that immune function is compromised. Chylous ascites and/or pleural effusions develop in 20 to 50 percent of patients. Therapy is principally nutritional with institution of a low-fat diet, high in medium-chain triglycerides. This serves to reduce lymphatic flow and the secondary complications of the lymphatic abnormality.

205. The answer is E (all). *(Alpert, N Engl J Med 285:185–189, 1971. Sabesin, N Engl J Med 290:944–950, 996–1002, 1974.)* Human hepatitis B (serum hepatitis) is associated with the hepatitis B antigen and can be identified by the presence of surface antigens, core antigens, or Dane particles, which are thought to be intact hepatitis B viruses. A prodrome of migratory arthritis or skin rash recently has been recognized and presumably is due to surface antigen-antibody immune complexes. Although traditionally associated with hepatitis A, oral-fecal transmission also has been linked to hepatitis B.

206. The answer is A (1, 2, 3). *(Goldman, N Engl J Med 293:20–23, 1975.)* Sulfasalazine (Azulfidine) is converted by bacteria in the colon into two active ingredients: 5-aminosalicylate and sulfapyridine. The mechanism for the drug's therapeutic action is unknown. It is most efficacious in the treatment of individuals who have ulcerative colitis and is currently thought to be of value but unproven efficacy in cases of Crohn's disease involving the small bowel. Adverse reactions can occur in patients as a result of allergic reactions, neutropenia and in those who are slow acetylators of sulfapyridine and thus develop toxic levels of this drug in their sera.

207. The answer is D (4). *(Petersdorf, ed 10. pp 1738–1752. Silverman, ed 3. pp 370–389.)* Crohn's disease (granulomatous colitis) characteristically is associated with transmural, granulomatous intestinal lesions that are discontinuous and can appear in both the small and large intestine. Although Crohn's disease first may appear as a rectal fissure or fistula, the rectum often is spared. Aphthous stomatitis is a common complaint in affected children. In relation to the general population, the risk of colonic carcinoma in affected individuals is increased but not nearly to the degree associated with ulcerative colitis.

208. The answer is E (all). *(Silverman, ed 3. pp 819–832. Sleisenger, ed 3. pp 1436–1450.)* Children who have cystic fibrosis can exhibit a wide range of gastrointestinal disorders: indeed, malabsorption in children is more likely to be due to cystic fibrosis than to any other cause. Hepatic lesions associated with cystic fibrosis include portal hypertension (often accompanied by varices and ascites), cirrhosis, and fatty disease. Among affected newborn infants, meconium ileus can lead to intestinal obstruction; obstruction in older children can occur for a variety of reasons. Gallbladder disorders associated with cystic fibrosis include congenital microgallbladder and cholelithiasis.

209. The answer is E (all). *(Silverman, ed 3. pp 347, 375, 389.)* Crohn's disease is a granulomatous disorder that can affect any area of the small or large intestine; another granulomatous disorder, cavitary pulmonary tuberculosis, can lead to ileocecal disease. Intestinal lesions of Schönlein-Henoch purpura can be caused by hemorrhage into the mucosal wall; almost any area of the gastrointestinal tract, however, can be similarly affected. *Yersinia enterocolitica* infection causes an acute gastroenteritis or a more persistent, localized disease involving the colon and distal ileum, often mimicking inflammatory bowel disease. Diagnosis may be confirmed by culture, serological titers, or both.

210. The answer is A (1, 2, 3). *(Silverman, ed 3. pp 158–161.)* Esophageal achalasia is a disease of unknown etiology characterized by the absence of peristalsis in the body of the esophagus and by failure of the lower esophageal sphincter (LES) to relax in response to swallowing. Histologically, there is degeneration of Auerbach's plexus and intraneural nerve cells. Motility patterns reveal elevated lower esophageal pressure with a failure to initiate neural relaxation of LES in response to swallowing. This should be differentiated from organic strictures of the lower esophagus. This disease is not associated with pseudoobstruction syndrome, which involves motor disorders of the small and large intestine as well as the esophagus.

211. The answer is E (all). *(Silverman, ed 3. pp 14, 15, 300, 888–897. Peters-dorf, ed 10. p 1735.)* Lactase is a disaccharidase localized in the brush border of the intestinal villous cells. It hydrolyzes lactose to its constituent monosaccharides, glucose and galactose. Intestinal lactase levels are usually normal at birth in all populations; however, lactase deficiency is a common genetically predetermined condition with an incidence reported to be 5 to 15 percent of the adult white population and 80 to 90 percent of adult blacks and orientals. Sucrose, also a disaccharide, is a nonreducing sugar composed of glucose and fructose that is hydrolyzed by the brush border enzyme sucrase. Lactase activity is not readily increased by the oral administration of substrate or the inclusion of lactose in the diet. The clinical symptoms of lactose malabsorption are due to the presence of osmotically active undigested lactose which may act to increase intestinal fluid volume, alter transit time, and produce the symptoms of abdominal cramps, distension, and, occasionally, watery diarrhea. Bacterial metabolism of the nonabsorbed carbohydrates in the colon to carbon dioxide and hydrogen may contribute to the clinical symptoms. Acquired lactase deficiency is often associated with conditions of the gastrointestinal tract that cause intestinal mucosal injury (e.g., sprue and reginal enteritis).

Diagnostic techniques for lactose intolerance include removal of the offending sugar with a reproduction of symptoms following an oral load (2 g/kg, maximum 50 g). This should be accompanied by the failure to demonstrate a rise in blood sugar of more than 300 mg/100 ml. Although the ingestion of even small amounts of lactose can be diagnostic if gastrointestinal symptoms occur, the measurement of breath hydrogen is more specific as it is not affected by glucose metabolism or gastric emptying. Similarly, an acidic stool pH in the presence of reducing substances would be diagnostic. Direct measurement of enzyme levels combined with histologic evaluation helps to differentiate an acquired (secondary versus primary) lactase deficiency in which the intestinal histology is normal.

212. The answer is B (1, 3). *(Silverman, ed 3. pp 21, 494–555.)* Obstructive jaundice (i.e., a direct-reacting bilirubin greater than 15 percent of the total) requires investigation in all infants. Cystic fibrosis and alpha₁-antitrypsin deficiency should be considered in the diagnostic evaluation of any child with these presenting findings. Other diseases to be excluded include galactosemia, tyrosinemia, and urinary tract or other infections, including toxoplasmosis, cytomegalovirus, rubella, syphilis, and herpesvirus. Ultrasound examination to rule out choledochal cyst may be included with an ^{131}I rose bengal or [99]technetium hepatic imindodiacetic acid (HIDA) scan to assess the patency of the biliary tree. Liver biopsy may show evidence of hepatitis and giant cell transformation both in cystic fibrosis and alpha₁-antitrypsin deficiency. These findings may differentiate these diseases from extrahepatic obstruction or biliary atresia, but they are not pathognomonic in themselves. The presence of diastase-resistant, periodic acid schiff (PAS) positive granules is reported but is not specific in alpha₁-antitrypsin deficiency alone. In contrast, infants who have Gilbert's syndrome or hypothyroidism present with an indirect hyperbilirubinemia and have normal liver biopsies.

213. The answer is A (1, 2, 3). *(Silverman, ed 3. pp 265–279.)* Hartnup disease, folic acid deficiency, and dermatitis herpetiformis all disrupt the intestinal phase of digestion. Hartnup disease is an inborn defect in the absorption by intestinal epithelial cells of the amino acids tryptophan and phenylalanine. Folate deficiency, either as a congenital disorder or in association with the malabsorption syndrome, is a sign of jejunal mucosal dysfunction. Dermatitis herpetiformis, which may be associated with celiac sprue, can lead to patchy distribution of flat areas of intestinal mucosa. Cystic fibrosis is principally a defect of pancreatic function and lipolysis; thus, it interferes with the intraluminal phase of digestion.

214. The answer is A (1, 2, 3). *(Silverman, ed 3. pp 814–835.)* The x-ray presented in the question shows a microcolon (disuse microcolon), which is characteristic of fetal intestinal obstruction; it requires prompt diagnosis and therapeutic management. Films of the abdomen are the first step in establishing the diagnosis and possible level of obstruction in an infant with abdominal distension and clinical evidence of obstruction. With meconium ileus or meconium peritonitis a characteristic "soap bubble" appearance in the right lower quadrant or evidence of intestinal perforation might be evident. Barium enema is then often required to establish the presence of microcolon and to differentiate between a volvulus and other less common abnormalities. Ileal atresia secondary to meconium inspissation, intestinal perforation, and meconium peritonitis, with its associated intraabdominal calcifications, are frequently associated with cystic fibrosis. These begin in utero and are accompanied by a secondary microcolon. Occasionally, a microcolon may be present when acute intestinal obstruction due to malrotation and volvulus occurs very early in life. Evidence by barium enema of abnormal placement or lack of fixation of the cecum can suggest this diagnosis. Obstruction in Down's syndrome (trisomy 21) infants also can be caused by jejunoileal atresia, which may be accompanied by malrotation.

Tracheoesophageal fistula with esophageal atresia is associated with polyhydramnios secondary to a failure to reabsorb swallowed amniotic fluid in utero. It does not lead to microcolon unless there is a complete intestinal obstruction. Hirschsprung's disease presents in the newborn period with a delayed passage of meconium but with a normal or increased diameter of the colon; occasionally, there is evidence of enterocolitis. A transition zone may be seen by barium enema, often with failure to clear the barium over the next 24 hours.

Surgery is almost always required to correct meconium ileus. However, occasionally a diatrizoate methylglucamine (Gastrografin) enema or infusion of mycolytic agents such as N-acetylcystein (5 to 10% solution) has been useful to relieve the obstruction, thus alleviating the need for an intestinal resection. Enzyme replacement is required in the therapy of the pancreatic insufficiency associated with cystic fibrosis.

215. The answer is C (2, 4). *(Silverman, ed 3. p 272. Behrman, ed 12. 933–934.)* Symptoms of celiac disease, which include chronic vomiting and diarrhea, irritability, and failure to grow, most commonly present during the first two years of life. Small bowel x-rays of affected children often show thickened and coarse mucosal folds and dilatation of the intestine; small-bowel biopsy can show severely abnormal morphology. Celiac disease, an inherited condition in which the symptoms of malabsorption may occur sporadically within a family, is characterized by an intolerance to gluten. Treatment of affected children with a gluten-free diet is effective; however, removal of the offending agent is insufficient to establish the diagnosis. Histological recovery after removal of gluten is required, and on occasion it may be necessary to demonstrate recurrence of injury with gluten challenge. Proposed mechanisms for the initiation of injury include the absence of an intracellular or brush border peptidase, which renders the individual unable to digest gluten, and an immunologically mediated mechanism which involves the recognition of gluten as an offending agent. Histological features include an abnormal surface epithelium with loss of columnar cells, shortened villi, and elongation of crypts. While these are not specific for gluten-sensitive enteropathy, they are histologically consistent. Granuloma formation is not seen in celiac disease, nor is a pronounced eosinophilic inflammatory component. Treatment always involves gluten withdrawal and may also include a lactose-free diet if sufficient mucosal damage has occurred. Corticosteroids are reserved for use in acute celiac crises and in supportive management.

The histopathology of some other diarrheal diseases is as follows: ulcerative colitis does not involve the small intestine, and the small bowel biopsy in cystic fibrosis is normal. In lymphangiectasia the biopsy shows dilated lymphatics with a normal mucosa. In primary agammaglobulinemia there is an absence of plasma cells and a variety of histological abnormalities, particularly when complicated by giardiasis, malnutrition, or both. In congenital lactase deficiency, the small bowel biopsy is normal, and the diagnosis is established by enzyme analysis.

216–220. The answers are: 216-A, 217-C, 218-C, 219-C, 220-B. *(Rudolph, ed 17. pp 616–620.)* Non-A, non-B hepatitis has been found to be the most common cause of posttransfusion hepatitis since the advent of sensitive screening methods for hepatitis B surface antigen in transfused blood. Current estimates for the prevalence of non-A, non-B hepatitis as a cause of transfusion-related hepatitis range between 50 to 90 percent of all cases. Persistence of an infectious agent or agents has been documented in both diseases. These are both transmissible to an animal model. Chronic hepatitis occurs commonly with non-A, non-B hepatitis, as well as hepatitis B. Recent studies have demonstrated the efficacy and safety of a vaccine for hepatitis B; however, no vaccine is available for non-A, non-B hepatitis at the current time, nor has an identifiable agent(s) been isolated.

221–225. The answers are: 221-B, 222-A, 223-B, 224-C, 225-A. *(Silverman, ed 3. pp 700–711, 714–716.)* Wilson's disease, an autosomal recessive genetic disorder, is characterized by the defective metabolism of copper. Copper deposition particularly affects the brain — causing tremors, dystonia, and personality changes, and the liver — causing portal hypertension and postnecrotic cirrhosis among other conditions. Hemolysis can lead to recurrent jaundice and anemia. Renal defects, which are associated with glycosuria and aminoaciduria, often occur. Wilson's disease usually appears clinically in individuals between the ages of 6 and 20 years. Adminisration of D-penicillamine (Cuprimine) has been therapeutically helpful.

Alpha₁-antitrypsin deficiency, which has an autosomal codominant mode of inheritance, can cause chronic liver disease in infants and may give rise in adults to gradually developing dyspnea as a result of panacinar emphysema, early symptoms of which can appear in childhood. Jaundice can develop in affected infants during the first weeks of life; histologic examination of the liver shows intralobular bile stasis, perilobular fibrosis, and other abnormalities. Postnecrotic cirrhosis develops later. Management includes symptomatic treatment and genetic counseling.

226–230.   The answers are: 226-B, 227-B, 228-E, 229-C, 230-B. *(Silverman, ed 3. pp 455–465.)* All of the disorders listed in the question cause gastrointestinal polyposis. Peutz-Jeghers syndrome, which is inherited as an autosomal dominant trait, is characterized by the presence of hamartomatous polyps, especially in the small intestine but also occasionally in the stomach and colon. The most striking extraintestinal manifestation of this disorder is lip or buccal pigmentation, which usually develops during infancy. Peutz-Jeghers polyposis rarely leads to carcinoma.

Gardner's syndrome, on the other hand, is characterized by adenomatous polyps that frequently undergo malignant degeneration. This autosomal dominant disorder occurs mainly in the colon. In affected children under the age of ten years, the condition may appear first as a fibromatous mass or epidermoid cyst involving skin or soft tissue.

Isolated juvenile polyps occur as a benign, nonheritable condition typically associated with pedunculated inflammatory polyps that usually occur within 25 cm of the anus. Juvenile polyposis of the colon, in contrast, is an inherited condition (the mode of inheritance is unknown) causing large numbers of juvenile polyps to appear in the intestine. Neither disorder is associated with malignant degeneration. Although children having juvenile polyposis of the colon may have other congenital anomalies, children with juvenile polyps usually do not.

Lymphoid polyposis (nodular lymphoid hyperplasia) can affect both the small and the large intestine. In cases where the appearance of the submucosal nodules, which are composed of lymphoid follicles, is confined to the small intestine, infection with *Giardia lamblia* may be an etiologic factor. Lymphoid polyposis is associated neither with intestinal carcinoma nor with extraintestinal manifestations. Whether this condition is inherited is not known.

The Urinary Tract

Julie R. Ingelfinger

DIRECTIONS: Each question below contains five suggested answers. Choose the **one best** response to each question.

231. A three-year-old girl has a fever and foul-smelling urine. Urine culture reveals greater than 10^5 *Escherichia coli*/mm^3 sensitive to all antibiotics tested. When she is later studied with voiding cystourethrography, grade I reflux is found. All of the following steps in management would be appropriate EXCEPT to

(A) put her on the schedule for cystoscopy
(B) place her on prophylactic antibiotic therapy
(C) institute double micturition at bedtime
(D) place her on a program of home dip-slide cultures
(E) schedule a radionuclide voiding cystourethrogram for six months hence

232. All of the following statements about enuretic children are true EXCEPT that

(A) about 1 percent of normal children are enuretic at age 15
(B) about 12 percent of five-year-old boys are bedwetters
(C) a familial pattern is common
(D) organic renal disease is more prevalent in enuretic children
(E) operant conditioning is often therapeutically helpful

233. The presence of drug-induced nephrotic syndrome should be suspected in a proteinuric patient who has received which of the following drugs?

(A) Tetracycline
(B) Streptomycin
(C) Trimethadione
(D) Diazepam
(E) Chlorambucil

234. An *Escherichia coli* colony count of 2000/mm^3 would be definite evidence of a urinary tract infection if the sampled urine

(A) has a specific gravity of 1.008
(B) has been taken from a catheterized bladder and has a specific gravity of 1.022
(C) is from an ileal-loop bag
(D) is from a suprapubic tap
(E) is the first morning sample

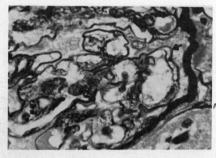

110 Pediatrics

235. A renal biopsy is performed on a 10-year-old boy with hematuria and proteinuria; a micrograph from the biopsy is shown below. The most likely diagnosis is

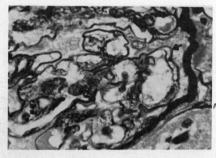

(A) segmental glomerulosclerosis
(B) postinfectious glomerulonephritis
(C) membranoproliferative glomerulonephritis
(D) crescenteric glomerulonephritis
(E) focal global glomerulosclerosis

236. A seven-year-old child develops acute renal failure. Laboratory studies are sent to differentiate prerenal, intrinsic, and obstructive renal failure. Urine and plasma osmolality (Osm), sodium (Na^+), urea, creatinine (Cr) are sent. With these, renal failure index (RFI) and fractional sodium excretion (FE_{Na+}) are calculated. Which of the following are most suggestive of prerenal failure?

(A) $U_{Osm} = 320$; $U_{Osm}/P_{Osm} = 1.0$; $U_{urea}/P_{urea} = 7.0$
(B) $U_{Na+} = 51$ meq/L; RFI = 1.2; $FE_{Na+} = 1.2$
(C) $U_{Osm} = 563$; $U_{urea}/P_{urea} = 8.6$; $FE_{Na+} = .9$
(D) $U_{Osm} = 480$; $U_{Na+} = 40$; $U_{urea}/P_{urea} = 7.8$
(E) $FE_{Na+} = 2.1$; $U_{Cr}/P_{Cr} = 18$; RFI = 2.7

237. An eight-year-old girl has a glomerular filtration rate of 100 ml/min per 1.73 m². Her urine specific gravity has never exceeded 1.010. These laboratory values could be associated with all of the following conditions EXCEPT

(A) diabetes insipidus
(B) sickle cell anemia
(C) childhood nephrosis
(D) nephrocalcinosis
(E) pyelonephritis

238. A blood pressure of 120/80 mmHg is within normal values for children of all of the following ages EXCEPT

(A) four years
(B) seven years
(C) ten years
(D) twelve years
(E) fifteen years

239. The cells shown below were seen on microscopic examination of a bacteriologically sterile urine specimen. The differential diagnosis should include all of the following conditions EXCEPT

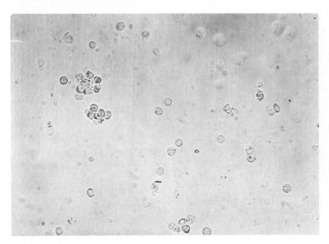

(A) renal tuberculosis
(B) systemic lupus erythematosus
(C) interstitial nephritis
(D) Potter's syndrome
(E) Kawasaki disease

240. An exogenous substance that is used to measure glomerular filtration rate should be

(A) physiologically active
(B) capable of binding with plasma proteins
(C) freely filterable at the glomerulus
(D) secreted by the renal tubule
(E) reabsorbed by the renal tubule

241. In lupus nephritis the glomeruli are the main sites of injury. All of the following may occur in lupus nephritis EXCEPT that

(A) one form of lupus nephritis may sometimes show transition to another
(B) mesangial widening and mesangial IgG and C3 deposits on renal biopsy are usually associated with hematuria and proteinuria
(C) the most serious and active type of lupus nephritis is diffuse proliferative lupus nephritis
(D) membranous lupus nephritis rarely, if ever, responds to treatment
(E) glomerular sclerosis may occur in all forms of lupus nephritis

242. The child shown in the photograph below most likely has

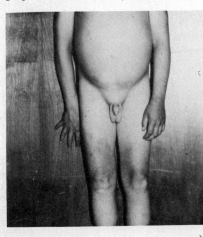

(A) cystinosis
(B) polycystic kidneys
(C) diabetes insipidus
(D) acute poststreptococcal glomerulonephritis
(E) nephrosis

243. A previously healthy six-year-old white boy develops acute renal failure. The pathologic processes in his illness may include all of the following EXCEPT

(A) obstructive uropathy
(B) acute papillary necrosis
(C) renal arterial occlusion
(D) myoglobinuria
(E) acute glomerulonephritis

244. All of the following statements about hypospadias are true EXCEPT that

(A) it is the most common penile anomaly
(B) it should not be repaired in infancy
(C) it is associated with chordee, more apparent on erection
(D) it is associated with meatal stenosis, inguinal hernia and undescended testes
(E) it demands radiographic evaluation to detect lower urinary tract problems

245. A ten-year-old boy comes to the emergency room complaining of flank pain. A flat-plate x-ray taken at that time is shown below. The findings exhibited by the x-ray could represent all of the following types of urinary stones EXCEPT

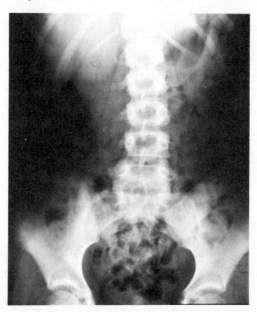

(A) cystine
(B) uric acid
(C) calcium phosphate
(D) calcium oxalate
(E) magnesium ammonium sulfate

246. A child who has vomited and had diarrhea for two days is brought to the emergency room for evaluation. No blood loss has occurred. Serum sodium level is reported to be 138 meq/L. This child, who weighed 10 kg (22 lb) last week, now weighs 9 kg (19.8 lb). The best therapy would be infusion of

(A) Ringer's lactate, 100 ml over two hours, followed by normal saline with 40 meq/L of potassium, 500 ml over sixteen hours, and 5% dextrose in quarter-normal saline, 1400 mml over the next eight hours

(B) Ringer's lactate, 200 ml over one to two hours, followed by 5% dextrose in quarter-normal saline, 800 ml over the next eight hours, and 1000 ml over the following sixteen hours

(C) whole blood, 100 ml over 30 minutes, followed by 5% dextrose in quarter-normal saline, 1800 ml over the following 20 to 24 hours

(D) plasma, 100 ml, followed by 5% dextrose in one-sixth-normal saline, 1900 ml over 16 hours

(E) plasma, 200 ml, followed by 5% dextrose in water, 1800 ml over 18 hours

247. A seven-year-old boy suffers multiple injuries as a result of blunt abdominal trauma. All of the following statements concerning the proper assessment and treatment of the injury are true EXCEPT that

(A) most renal injuries can be managed nonoperatively

(B) major vascular injuries require rapid surgical intervention

(C) rupture of a full bladder is uncommon

(D) traumatic hematocele requires surgical exploration and repair

(E) prompt surgical repair is needed for most ureteral injuries

248. A three-year-old boy develops edema and proteinuria. His serum cholesterol level is 322 mg/100 ml, and his serum albumin level is 1.9 g/100 ml. The likelihood that he has minimal-change nephrotic syndrome is about

(A) 10 percent

(B) 25 percent

(C) 40 percent

(D) 65 percent

(E) 80 percent

249. Funduscopic examination of a thirteen-year-old girl shows general and focal arteriolar narrowing. A hemorrhage is observed in the left retina, and sclerosis is present. Her blood pressure is 180/110 mmHg. This girl would be likely to exhibit all of the following symptoms or signs EXCEPT

(A) isolated facial nerve palsy
(B) headache
(C) hyporeflexia
(D) nocturnal wakening
(E) left ventricular hypertrophy

250. A ten-month-old child has diarrhea and is dehydrated by an estimated 10 percent. Laboratory analysis reveals a serum sodium level of 162 meq/L. The clinical sign or symptom that would be LEAST likely to accompany these findings would be

(A) increased reflexes
(B) impaired mental status
(C) marked thirst
(D) marked loss of circulatory volume
(E) doughy skin

251. Hereditary onychoosteodysplasia is the diagnosis reached in a baby with all of the following abnormalities EXCEPT

(A) ptosis
(B) sensorineural deafness
(C) thumbnail ridges
(D) renal disease
(E) flexion contractures

252. The photomicrograph shown below of a urine specimen from a seven-year-old child is LEAST likely to support a diagnosis of

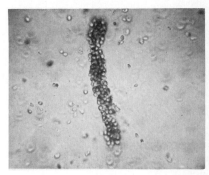

(A) systemic lupus erythematosus
(B) acute poststreptococcal glomerulonephritis
(C) Berger disease
(D) membranous glomerulopathy
(E) mesangiocapillary glomerulonephritis

253. During the first year of a child's life, all of the following parameters of renal function increase EXCEPT

(A) glomerular filtration rate
(B) nephron number
(C) renal plasma flow
(D) tubular reabsorptive capacity
(E) tubular secretory capacity

254. A seven-year-old boy has crampy abdominal pain and a rash on the back of his legs and buttocks as well as on the extensor surfaces of his forearms. Laboratory analysis reveals proteinuria and microhematuria. He is most likely to be affected by

(A) systemic lupus erythematosus
(B) anaphylactoid purpura
(C) poststreptococcal glomeru-lonephritis
(D) polyarteritis nodosa
(E) dermatomyositis

DIRECTIONS: Each question below contains four suggested answers of which *one or more* is correct. Choose the answer:

A	if	**1, 2, and 3**	are correct
B	if	**1 and 3**	are correct
C	if	**2 and 4**	are correct
D	if	**4**	is correct
E	if	**1, 2, 3, and 4**	are correct

255. The angiogram below is from a 12-year-old boy who has large kidneys. Findings on the x-ray are consistent with

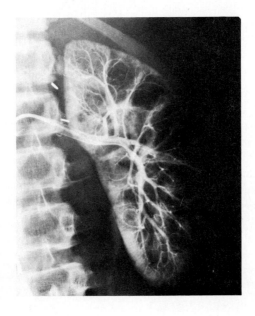

(1) multicystic renal dysplasia
(2) nephronophthisis
(3) megacalyx
(4) adult-type polycystic disease

SUMMARY OF DIRECTIONS

A	B	C	D	E
1,2,3 only	1,3 only	2,4 only	4 only	All are correct

256. Proximal renal tubular acidosis (RTA) can occur in association with which of the following?

(1) Obstructive uropathy
(2) Amphotericin B administration
(3) Ehlers-Danlos syndrome
(4) Lead poisoning

257. Correct statements concerning nephrogenic diabetes insipidus include which of the following?

(1) Most North American patients are of common descent
(2) It is probably inherited by an X-linked recessive mode
(3) It is a likely consequence of an enzymatic or biochemical renal tubular abnormality
(4) It is usually diagnosed at birth

258. Shunt nephritis typically has

(1) red blood cell casts
(2) decreased C3 level
(3) hypertension
(4) positive urine culture

259. The onset of chronic renal failure is likely to be associated with which of the following findings?

(1) Growth retardation
(2) Oliguria
(3) Anorexia
(4) Hypotonia

260. The findings one might expect in a six-year-old boy with brown urine and healing impetigo include which of the following?

(1) Hypertension
(2) Dyspnea
(3) Periorbital edema
(4) Hepatomegaly

261. A percutaneous kidney biopsy of a child who has steroid-dependent nephrosis should NOT be performed if that child also has which of the following complications?

(1) Single kidney
(2) Pyelonephritis
(3) Dysplastic kidneys
(4) Hypertension

262. For the last three months, a child, whose x-ray is shown below, has been treated with dihydrotachysterol, 0.25 mg/day. The condition depicted in this child's x-ray would be compatible with which of the following conditions?

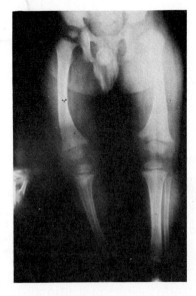

(1) Acidemia
(2) A serum phosphate level of 2.1 mg/100 ml
(3) A blood urea nitrogen level of 150 mg/100 ml
(4) A positive family history

263. An arteriogram of an eight-year-old girl who has hypertension is shown below. Findings illustrated in the arteriogram could be the result of

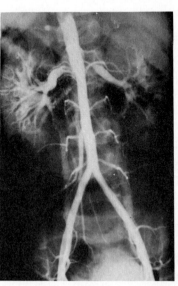

(1) fibromuscular dysplasia
(2) von Recklinghausen's disease
(3) tumorous impingement
(4) arteriovenous malformation

264. An 11-year-old girl repeatedly has first morning urines brought to your office with concentrations between 400 and 700 mOsm/kg H_2O. Diagnoses to be considered in her subsequent evaluation include

(1) chronic renal failure
(2) compulsive water drinking
(3) sickle cell disease
(4) nephrogenic diabetes insipidus (NDI)

SUMMARY OF DIRECTIONS

A	B	C	D	E
1,2,3 only	1,3 only	2,4 only	4 only	All are correct

---

265. A six-year-old girl is brought to the emergency room because her urine is red. Examination with Hemastix is negative. Possible causes of the red color of the girl's urine include

(1) ingestion of blackberries
(2) ingestion of beets
(3) phenolphthalein catharsis
(4) presence of myoglobin

266. Hemolytic uremic syndrome can be described by which of the following statements?

(1) It commonly is preceded by infection
(2) It is characterized by development of acute renal failure
(3) Children five years of age or less are most often affected
(4) Blacks are affected more often than whites

267. A 14-year-old boy who has renal dysplasia develops a urinary tract infection. His serum creatinine is reported to be 6.2 mg/100 ml. Which of the following antibiotics, as possible treatment for the boy's infection, would require dosage alteration in this situation?

(1) Ampicillin
(2) Amoxicillin
(3) Gentamicin
(4) Clindamycin

268. A 16-year-old girl, who has sickle cell disease and red-colored urine, undergoes intravenous pyelography. Her pyelogram, shown below, provides evidence of

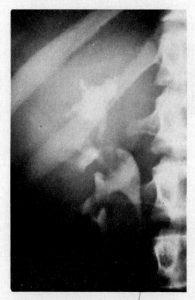

(1) a central papillary filling defect
(2) radiolucent cysts
(3) renal infarction
(4) renal stones

269. Abdominal ultrsasound is a useful diagnostic tool that is able to

(1) localize kidneys for renal biopsy
(2) determine whether or not a renal mass is cystic
(3) differentiate multicystic kidney from hydronephrosis
(4) differentiate hydronephrosis from urinomas, hematomas, or lymphoceles

270. Congenital nephrosis is characterized by

(1) circulating immune complexes
(2) frequent gross hematuria
(3) responsiveness to steroid therapy
(4) a high familial incidence

DIRECTIONS: The groups of questions below consist of lettered choices followed by several numbered items. For each numbered item select the **one** lettered choice with which it is **most** closely associated. Each lettered choice may be used once, more than once, or not at all.

Questions 271–275

For each condition listed below, match the category to which it belongs.

(A) Primary renal tubular defect
(B) Developmental structural abnormality
(C) Metabolic disorder leading to renal damage
(D) Multisystem disorder
(E) Primary renal disease with multiple renal manifestations
(F) No renal involvement

271. Cystinuria A

272. Wilson's disease C

273. Alport syndrome E

274. Prune belly syndrome D

275. Crossed, fused ectopia B

Questions 276–280

For each diagnosis that follows, select the mode of inheritance with which it is associated.

(A) Autosomal dominant
(B) Autosomal recessive
(C) X-linked dominant
(D) X-linked recessive
(E) None of the above

276. Hypophosphatemic rickets C

277. Infantile polycystic disease B

278. Systemic lupus erythematosus E

279. Nephropathic cystinosis B

280. Adult-type polycystic disease A

The Urinary Tract

Answers

231. The answer is A. *(Behrman, ed 12. pp 1367–1372, 1396–1398.)* Cystoscopy is no longer deemed necessary in children with minimal grades of reflux. Furthermore, urethral calibration and dilatation are not helpful in protecting against subsequent infections. Prophylactic antibiotic therapy at bedtime, or twice daily, may minimize reinfection and should be continued while there is reflux. The majority of children with reflux will respond to nonoperative management. Reevaluation of the urinary tract periodically is necessary in order to follow the course of reflux, especially in a child under age five who is particularly vulnerable to developing renal scars.

232. The answer is D. *(Behrman, ed 12. p 1381.)* Daytime wetting is rare in children who have reached the age of six. However, at this age at least 8 percent of girls and 12 percent of boys are nocturnally enuretic. A careful history should be taken and a physical examination, including urinalysis, should be performed on children whose enuresis has persisted to the age of six. Organic disease is no more prevalent in enuretic than in other children, and blood urea nitrogen and serum creatinine studies and intravenous urography are warranted only if there is evidence of an organic lesion. Treatment, which should attempt to reassure affected children and their parents, can include behavior modification techniques and the use of imipramine (Tofranil).

233. The answer is C. *(Behrman, ed 12. p 1382.)* Drug-related nephrotic syndrome has been described in connection with the use of trimethadione, penicillamine, tolbutamide, and certain heavy metals. A variety of allergenic causes, including Hymenoptera stings, pollens, insect bites, and snakebites, also have been implicated as etiologic agents. Nephrosis can develop in conjunction with malignancy and diseases such as amyloidosis.

234. The answer is D. *(Behrman, ed 12. pp 1369–1370.)* No bacteria at all should grow in a properly obtained urine sample from a suprapubic tap or from retrograde catheterization of the upper urinary tract. Infected urine of low specific gravity often contains less than 10^5 colonies/mm^3, but a count as low as 2000/mm^3 would be unlikely. First-morning urine usually is concentrated, and a higher colony count thus would be expected. Ileal-loop bags are usually contaminated. Depending on technique, bladder catheterization of a normal person may produce urine with a low organism count.

235. The answer is C. *(Behrman, ed 12. pp 1328–1329.)* Membranoproliferative glomerulonephritis, a chronic, diffuse, proliferative nephritis, occurs in two main forms that are clinically indistinguishable. The micrograph shown in the question depicts type I membranoproliferative glomerulonephritis (MPGN type I) with interposition of mesangial matrix between the basement membrane and the endothelial layer. Subendothelial deposits are also seen. Type I MPGN is more common than type II, which is called "dense deposit disease" because denseappearing deposits occur within the basement membrane. Complement abnormalities are usually found in both MPGN type I and type II. In type I C3 is variably decreased and depression of C1q and C4 are often seen. In type II C3 is said to be more persistently decreased, suggesting alternative pathway activation. Progressive renal failure may occur in either form.

236. The answer is C. *(Behrman, ed 12. p 1359.)* In prerenal failure, urinary sodium is usually low, as reflected here in choice C where the fractional excretion of sodium is under 1. In intrinsic and obstructive acute renal failure it is usually higher, and FE_{Na+} is greater than 1. In prerenal failure, tubular function is relatively preserved, and urinary concentration is better than in other forms of acute renal failure, which is reflected by U_{Osm} over 500 mOsm/kg H_2O and U_{Osm}/P_{Osm} greater than 1.3. U_{Cr}/P_{Cr} is usually more than 40, and U_{urea}/P_{urea} greater than 8 for similar reasons. Differentiating prerenal from other forms of acute renal failure is important because therapy differs.

237. The answer is C. *(Behrman, ed 12. pp 1311, 1323, 1347, 1355, 1372.)* In individuals affected by childhood nephrosis, there is a reduced ability to excrete a free water load; thus, urine is highly concentrated. Sickle-cell patients have isothenuria, probably due to the sickling of erythrocytes in the vasa recta. Patients who have diabetes insipidus cannot concentrate their urine, either because of a lack of vasopressin (central diabetes insipidus) or an unresponsiveness to vasopressin (nephrogenic diabetes insipidus). Because patients who have pyelonephritis have interstitial tubular damage, they may not be able to concentrate urine.

238. The answer is A. *(Behrman, ed 12. p 1101.)* Average blood pressure tends to increase with age. Thus, a value of 120/80 mmHg, clearly acceptable for most children, is in the hypertensive range for children in the first few years of life. In the newborn period, a systolic pressure above 90 mmHg is considered hypertensive.

239. The answer is D. *(Behrman, ed 12. pp 580, 1337, 1372–1373, 1382–1383.)* In Potter's syndrome, the kidneys are absent; consequently, pyuria cannot be present. Potter's syndrome is a lethal abnormality that may be suspected at birth by the presence of oligohydramnios, a wizened appearance, and a characteristic wide semicircular fold of skin that extends downward and laterally from the inner canthus of both eyes. There may also be pulmonary hypoplasia. Sterile pyuria, as evidenced by the depicted white blood cells, may occur in febrile illness dehydration, acute nephritides, renal cystic disease, toxic nephropathy, and renal transplant rejection, as well as in the other disorders listed in the question.

240. The answer is C. *(Behrman, ed 12. pp 1303–1304, 1312–1313.)* If an exogenous substance is capable of being metabolized, bound by plasma proteins, or secreted or reabsorbed by the renal tubule, it will not measure glomerular function adequately. With current radiologic techniques, it is possible to perform glomerular-filtration-rate studies with isotopes such as ^{51}Cr-ethylenediaminotetraacetate (^{51}Cr-EDTA) or ^{125}I-iothalamate. Nonradiolabeled substances such as inulin, cyanocobalamin, and mannitol may also be used.

241. The answer is B. *(Behrman, ed 12. pp 1336–1337.)* There are five forms of systemic lupus erythematosus nephritis: mesangial, focal proliferative, diffuse proliferative, membranous, and interstitial. Of these, mesangial lupus nephritis is often present with a normal urinalysis. It has been hypothesized that all forms of lupus nephritis begin with mesangial changes such as widening, hypercellularity, and deposition of IgG and C^3. Focal proliferative lupus nephritis generally has a benign prognosis, wheras diffuse proliferative nephritis may progress quickly to renal failure if not treated. Membranous lupus nephritis responds minimally, if at all, to therapy but progresses slowly.

242. The answer is E. *(Behrman, ed 12. pp 1323–1324, 1332.)* Physical findings of individuals who have nephrosis usually stem from edema, which may progress to generalized edema (anasarca). The edema is typically pitting and shifts with position. Although edema may occur in association with acute nephritis, it usually is less marked than in nephrosis. The large abdomens of patients who have polycystic kidney disease are not edematous. Cystinosis and diabetes insipidus do not cause edema.

243. The answer is B. *(Behrman, ed 12. p 1355.)* Acute and widespread glomerular injury is a common source of acute renal failure in children. Acute glomerulonephritis, rapidly progressive glomerulonephritis, and hemolyticuremic syndrome are all associated with widespread glomerular injury. In children, acute tubular necrosis and bilateral cortical necrosis may also occur. In a white child, acute papillary necrosis would be most unlikely, as this entity is associated with sickle cell disease.

244. The answer is E. *(Behrman, ed 12. pp 1392–1393.)* Hypospadias occurs in 0.1 to 0.33 percent of live births. If the degree of hypospadias is mild, radiographic or panendoscopic examination is very unlikely to find lower urinary tract anomalies, and neither is recommended. Though hypospadias should be repaired before a child enters school, repair in infancy is not recommended. Management should be individualized, as a one- or two-stage repair may be needed. The psychological effects must be given careful attention.

245. The answer is B. *(Behrman, ed 12. pp 1376–1377.)* Xanthine stones and, to a lesser degree, uric acid stones are radiolucent and therefore do not show up on flat-plate x-rays. When contrast material is used, however, radiolucent stones show up well (as filling defects), whereas radiopaque stones often blend in with the x-ray dye. Although 50 to 60 percent of urinary tract stones in children are idiopathic, a full metabolic workup is indicated to rule out the presence of underlying disease.

246. The answer is B. *(Behrman, ed 12. pp 228–249.)* The sodium deficit of the child described in the question is probably 8 to 10 meq/kg, or a total of 80 to 100 meq. Sodium maintenance would require the infusion of another 10 to 20 meq/24 hours. Use of normal saline would provide too much sodium for the child described, whereas one-sixth-normal saline would supply too little. Administration of whole blood or packed red blood cells is rarely needed in the absence of blood loss; also, plasma and blood both carry a finite risk of subsequent serum hepatitis. Potassium should not be added to intravenous solutions until adequate urine output has been established.

247. The answer is C. *(Behrman, ed 12. pp 1401–1402.)* Because it is an abdominal organ in children, the bladder, especially when full, is often ruptured by blunt trauma and lower abdominal wounds. Though small bladder tears may be treated conservatively by catheter drainage, surgical exploration is likely to be needed. Extensive urethral injuries may require surgical drainage of periurethral hematoma, primary surgical repair, or even urinary diversion procedures. Most ureteral injuries require prompt surgical intervention, though such injuries are rare because of the protected position of the ureter. A retrograde cystourethrogram and intravenous urography may be helpful, especially with pelvic fracture or suspected renal trauma.

248. The answer is E. *(Behrman, ed 12. p 1324.)* The patient described is of the sex and age most typical for minimal-change nephrotic syndrome, which accounts for about 80 percent of all cases of idiopathic nephrotic syndrome of childhood. The presence of highly selective proteinuria, normal renal function, a normal urinary sediment, and normal blood pressure further increases the likelihood of minimal-change disease. Histologically, the glomeruli of children affected by minimal-change nephrotic diseases are normal, except for smudging of epithelial foot processes.

249. The answer is C. *(Behrman, ed 12. pp 1195–1200.)* Important clinical signs of hypertension in children may include headache, dizziness, visual disturbances, irritability, and nocturnal wakening. Hypertensive encephalopathy may be preceded or accompanied by vomiting, hyperreflexia, ataxia, and focal or generalized seizures. Facial palsy may be the sole manifestation of severe hypertension. When marked fundal changes are present or when there are signs of vascular compromise, emergency treatment of the accompanying hypertension is warranted. Such hypertensive individuals require immediate hospitalization for diagnosis and therapy.

250. The answer is D. *(Behrman, ed 12. pp 228–249.)* Due to relatively good preservation of circulatory volume, patients who have hypertonic (hypernatremic) dehydration may look stable clinically. However, because the central nervous system is especially liable to insult, therapy must be approached cautiously. Brain edema, for example, can result from the too rapid administration of dilute solution; too much sodium, on the other hand, may increase the danger of brain hemorrhage. Careful and gradual replacement therapy is needed in most cases.

251. The answer is B. *(Behrman, ed 12. p 1354.)* Hereditary onychoosteodysplasia (nail-patella syndrome) is an autosomal dominant constellation of abnormalities closely linked to ABO blood groups. Affected individuals typically have multiple bony abnormalities such as absent or hypoplastic patellae, hypoplasia of proximal radial heads, talipes equinovarus, and iliac horns. Ocular abnormalities including glaucoma, microcornea, strabismus, abnormal iris pigmentation, and ptosis are typical. Hypoplasia, absence, ridging, or flatness of nails, particularly of the index fingers and thumbs, are frequent. Joint contractures, of elbows in particular, are seen. Renal disease is present and may progress to renal failure in about 20 percent of affected individuals. Proteinuria is the most common presentation of renal disease, with mild urinary concentrating defect or microhematuria as well in some patients.

252 The answer is D. *(Behrman, ed 12. pp 1327–1328, 1330, 1332, 1335, 1336–1338.)* The figure accompanying the question depicts a red blood cell cast characteristically found in the urine of patients with glomerular disease. Important exceptions include the minimal lesion form of the hephrotic syndrome (lipoid nephrosis) and membranous glomerulopathy. In these, the urine contains large amounts of protein and hyaline casts but few red blood cells.

253. The answer is B. *(Behrman, ed 12. pp 1307–1308.)* The kidneys of a newborn infant already contain their full complement of nephrons. However, glomerular filtration rate and renal plasma flow steadily increase to close to normal adult values (corrected for surface area) by the end of the first year of life. Infants have a relatively low rate of sodium reabsorption, which increases proportionally as body weight increases. The secretion of substances such as paraaminohippuric acid also increases during the first year of life.

254. The answer is B. *(Behrman, ed 12 pp 575–579, 581, 605–606, 1338–1340.)* The rash of anaphylactoid purpura most often involves extensor surfaces of the extremities; the face, soles, palms, and trunk are rarely affected. Both systemic lupus etrythematosus and dermatomyositis often are accompanied by typical facial rashes (butterfly and heliotrope, respectively). Individuals who have polyarteritis usually do not present with a rash. The scarlatiniform rash characteristic of streptococcal infections generally does not coincide with the development of poststreptococcal nephritis; impetiginous lesions, however, may still be present.

255. The answer is D (4). *(Behrman, ed 12. pp 1353–1354, 1357, 1375, 1385.)* The radiograph that accompanies the question shows the splayed-out calyces and large kidneys typical of adult-type polycystic kidneys, which can first appear in childhood. Multicystic kidneys are often unilateral; bilateral involvement in a 12-year-old child would be unlikely to be associated with the level of renal function pictured in the angiogram. Individuals who have nephronophthisis usually have normal or small-sized kidneys. Megacalyx is a rare entity in which the calyces appear large and can be mistaken for cysts; however, the renal cortex is normal.

256. The answer is D (4). *(Behrman, ed 12. p 1344.)* Renal tubular acidosis (RTA) is characterized by normal anion gap metabolic acidosis with hyperchloremia. Though glomerular filtration rate is usually normal, plasma bicarbonate is not maintained either due to defective urinary acidification (distal RTA) or impaired reabsorption of bicarbonate (proximal RTA). Though both proximal and distal forms of RTA may occur as primary entities, a variety of substances and diseases are associated with either one or the other form. For example, proximal RTA is associated with heavy metal poisoning, outdated tetracycline, renovascular accidents in the newborn period, cystinosis, Lowe syndrome, and Wilson disease. Distal RTA is associated with amphotericin B exposure, Ehlers-Danlos syndrome, toluene exposure, lithium salt administration, and other entities.

257. The answer is A (1, 2, 3). *(Behrman, ed 12. pp 1347–1349.)* Nephrogenic diabetes insipidus is a hereditary congenital disorder in which the urine is hypotonic and produced in large volumes because the kidneys fail to respond to antidiuretic hormone. Most North American patients thus involved are descendants of Ulster Scots who came to Nova Scotia in 1761 on the ship Hopewell. Males are primarily affected, apparently through an X-linked recessive mode, though there can be a variable expression in heterozygous females. The defect is unknown, but the disorder is felt to result from primary unresponsiveness of the distal tubule and collecting duct to vasopressin. Although the condition is present at birth, the diagnosis is often not made until several months later when excessive thirst, frequent voidings of large volumes of dilute urine, dehydration, and failure to thrive become obvious. Maintenance of adequate fluid intake and diet and use of saluretic drugs are the bases of therapy of this incurable disease.

258. The answer is A (1, 2, 3). *(Behrman, ed 12. p 1336.)* With infected ventriculoatrial (VA) shunts, as well as in subacute bacterial endocarditis and osteomyelitis, a proliferative glomerulonephritis may occur. Immune complex glomerulonephritis with IgG or IgM plus antigens of the bacteria has been postulated to be involved. Serum C3 is usually low. Typical presentation may include both nephrotic and nephritic features. Hematuria, proteinuria, and red blood cell casts are often seen in the urine. Urine culture is usually negative, wheras blood cultures are frequently positive. Azotemia and hypertension are uncommon.

259. The answer is B (1, 3). *(Behrman, ed 12. p 1363.)* Chronic renal failure (CRF) often has a gradual, even insidious, onset with vague complaints, including nausea, loss of appetite, fatigue, and headache. Decreased urinary concentrating ability is reflected by nocturia, polyuria, and polydipsia. Later in the course of CRF, declining urine volume may be seen. Growth failure may occur, and accompanying renal osteodystrophy may be reflected by bone or joint pain. Muscle cramps and paresthesias are common, but hypotonia is not.

260. The answer is E (all). *(Behrman, ed 12. pp 1331–1334.)* The most common form of acute glomerulonephritis involves the deposition of complement, immunoglobulin G, and properdin in glomeruli following a skin or throat infection with certain nephritogenic strains of group A β-hemolytic streptococci. Hematuria often colors the urine dark, and decreased urinary output may result in circulatory congestion and volume overload, which can induce dyspnea, periorbital edema, tachycardia, and hepatomegaly. Acute hypertension is common and may lead to headache, vomiting, and even encephalopathy with seizures. Congestive heart failure may occur.

261. The answer is E (all). *(Behrman, ed 12. p 1313.)* Hypertension increases the risk of bleeding after a percutaneous kidney biopsy and therefore should be controlled before a biopsy is performed. Patients who have single kidneys or renal dysplasis are at risk for loss of kidney function if they are subjected to closed renal biopsy. Septicemia can result from kidney biopsy of an individual affected by acute pyelonephritis. Although percutaneous kidney biopsy can be performed in the presence of mild edema, patients who have anasarca should first undergo diuresis.

262. The answer is C (2, 4). *(Behrman, ed 12. pp 1656–1657.)* Because the obviously rachitic bones revealed in the x-ray accompanying the question do not show hallmarks of renal osteodystrophy, neither an elevated level of blood urea nitrogen nor acidemia would be likely. Although the radiographic findings suggest nutritional rickets, a three-month course of dihydrotachysterol at the given doses would have been sufficient to cure a patient who has this disease. Thus, in view of the radiographic evidence and low serum phosphorus level, the likely diagnosis for the child described is vitamin D-resistant rickets, which also is called familiar hypophosphatemic rickets.

263. The answer is A (1, 2, 3). *(Behrman, ed 12. pp 1379–1380.)* Causes of renal artery stenosis include abnormalities of the renal vessel wall, external encroachment by tumor or cyst, and embolism. Revascularization by means of arterial repair, vascular grafts, and autotransplantation is essential if hypertension is severe. Renovascular hypertension has been reported in infants as well as in older children.

264. The answer is A (1, 2, 3). *(Behrman, ed 12. pp 1311, 1348.)* Children over age two years should have a first morning urine with a concentration of about 1100 mOsm (usual range: 870–1300). A variety of disorders impair renal concentrating ability including interstitial diseases, such as acute interstitial nephritis, and medullary injury, such as that associated with hypdronephrosis or sickle cell disease. NDI patients have decreased ability to concentrate their urine and would be unlikely to have urinary concentration greater than 150 mOsm/kg H_2O. With compulsive water drinking, not possible to control in an outpatient setting, a first morning urine may not be concentrated. Further testing should include other parameters of renal function and more specific tests of water and solute handling.

265. The answer is A (1, 2, 3). *(Behrman, ed 12. pp 1307–1308.)* A number of pH-dependent substances can impart a red color to urine. Use of phenolphthalein, a cathartic agent, or phenindione, an anticoagulant, can cause red urine; ingestion of blackberries or beets also may lead to red coloration ("beeturia"). Because myoglobin tests heme-positive in a Hemastix examination, myoglubinuria could not be the source of the red color of the urine of the girl described. Hematuria should be confirmed by dipstick testing as well as by microscopic examination of urinary sediment.

266. The answer is A (1, 2, 3). *(Behrman, ed 12. pp 1340–1343.)* Hemolytic uremic syndrome typically affects young children five years of age or less. The hallmarks of this disease, which often follows a viral-like gastrointestinal or upper respiratory tract illness, are severe hemolytic anemia, intravascular hemolysis, and platelet consumption that accompany acute renal failure. Hypertension, encephalopathy, and anuria also may occur. The syndrome seems to occur more frequently in whites than blacks.

267. The answer is A (1, 2, 3). *(Behrman, ed 12. p 1366.)* Many antibiotics require dosage alteration when administered to patients in renal failure. For this reason, it is best to avoid use of tetracyclines, methenamine, and nitrofurantoin completely. Major modification is required for gentamicin and other aminoglycosides. Penicillins, including ampicillin and amoxicillin, also require dosage modification. No dosage modification is needed with clindamycin therapy.

268. The answer is B (1, 3). *(Behrman, ed 12. p 1355. Vaughan, ed 11. p 1529.)* Papillary necrosis, a severe disorder affecting individuals who have sickle cell disease, may appear on an intravenous pyelogram as a central papillary filling defect or as distortion of a papilla. Renal infarction, brought on by bleeding, also can occur. If lots are present, hydronephrosis caused by obstruction may result. Neither stones nor cystic changes are characteristic features of sickle cell disease.

269. The answer is E (all). *(Behrman, ed 12. pp 1314, 1318.)* Renal ultrasound is noninvasive, and there is no unnecessary radiation exposure. Repeated studies are easily obtained for follow-up of problems. Renal ultrasound is especially helpful when kidneys cannot be visualized urographically. It is helpful in evaluating abdominal masses, especially in the newborn, and in examining transplanted kidneys. For example, renal ultrasound may be helpful in differentiating neoplasms from multicystic kidneys and hydronephrosis.

270. The answer is D (4). *(Behrman, ed 12. p 1329.)* Congenital nephrosis (infantile nephrosis), which occurs with an increased incidence among families having a history of the disease, is almost totally insensitive to any form of therapy. The characteristic lesion is cystic dilatation of the proximal tubules. Screening for elevated alpha-fetoprotein in maternal serum should be done in at-risk pregnancies.

271–275. The answers are: 271-A, 272-C, 273-E, 274-D, 275-B. *(Behrman, ed 12. pp 978, 1349–1352, 1375, 1391–1392.)* All of the conditions listed have some familial associations, although prune belly syndrome (triad syndrome) and crossed, fused ectopia also occur sporadically. Patients with cystinuria have a defect of amino acid transport in both renal tubules and the gastrointestinal tract that leads to renal calculi from cystine. Treatment consists of maintaining high urinary flow rate and alkalinizing the urine, both of which decrease stone formation. D-penicillamine may be effective in dissolving stones, as it forms a mixed disulfide of cysteine-penicillamine that is fifty times more soluble than cystine.

Patients with Wilson's disease also have a propensity to form stones and may have other renal problems such as hematuria and glycosuria.

In Alport syndrome, the most common inheritable renal disease, glomerular and tubular lesions both occur. Mean age of renal disease onset is six years, and end stage renal disease occurs in half of males before age 30. Women are not usually so severely affected and may have only mild urinary abnormalities. Deafness and ocular abnormalities occur in some kindreds.

Prune belly syndrome, which consists of the triad of absent abdominal musculature, cryptorchidism, and dysplasia of the urinary tract, often with megacystis-megaureter, usually presents in infancy because of the typical somatic features. The severity of renal involvement varies, with some patients developing chronic renal insufficiency.

Crossed, fused renal ectopia is generally not associated with clinical problems. However, the ectopic kidney may be more prone than a normally placed kidney to infection. If the ectopic kidney has an extopic ureter, there may be constant perineal wetness.

276–280. The answers are: 276-C, 277-B, 278-E, 279-B, 280-A. *(Behrman, ed 12. pp 430, 575–577, 1336–1338, 1356–1357, 1653–1654, 1656, 1660.)* All of the disorders listed in the question are clearly familiar except for systemic lupus erythematosus, which appears to result from a combination of environmental and genetic causes. Many current investigators believe that lupus may result from a viral infection in genetically predisposed individuals.

Hypophosphatemic rickets (vitamin D-resistant rickets) is characteristically inherited as an X-linked dominant trait. Affected males usually have a more severe form of this disease than affected females.

Children born with infantile polycystic kidney disease, an autosomal recessive disorder, often die in infancy from pulmonary disease or hypertension. Renal failure also may occur. Liver disease, the main source of later problems, can lead to portal hypertension, which often can be relieved by shunting procedures. Children who have infantile polycystic disease usually do not survive to 20 years of age.

Adult-type polycystic kidney disease, inherited in an autosomal-dominant fashion, is often seen in successive generations of the same family. If adult-type polycystic kidney disease is discovered in a family, siblings and parents should undergo intravenous urography or abdominal ultrasound studies.

Nephropathic cystinosis is an autosomal recessive disease in which affected patients develop renal failure by their early teens. Now that some individuals who have cystine storage disease are receiving renal allografts, the pathologic effects of cystine storage in tissues other than the kidney may become clinically important. Cystinosis should not be confused with cystinuria, which is characterized by nephrolithiasis.

The Neuromuscular System

Jerome S. Haller

DIRECTIONS: Each question below contains five suggested answers. Choose the **one best** response to each question.

281. A diagnosis of Tourette syndrome is based on the patient's history of

(A) a past history of encephalitis
(B) drug addiction
(C) repetitive writhing movements of the extremities
(D) positive response to methylphenidate
(E) brief, stereotypic movements of face and limbs

282. The virus causing subacute sclerosing panencephalitis is presumed to be which of the following?

(A) Rubella
(B) Epstein-Barr
(C) Herpes simplex
(D) Herpes zoster
(E) Measles virus

283. Neonatal seizures have several different clinical manifestations, the most common being "subtle" seizures. Tonic episodes, though less common, have a prognostically poorer outcome. Of the following, what might these episodes represent?

(A) Apneic spells
(B) Breath-holding spells
(C) Drug intoxication
(D) Decerebrate posturing
(E) None of the above

284. The most frequent complication of congenital rubella is believed to be

(A) cataracts
(B) microcephaly
(C) patent ductus arteriosus
(D) deafness
(E) thrombocytopenia

285. Which of the following aminoacidopathies is associated with acute infantile hemiplegia?

(A) Phenylketonuria
(B) Homocystinuria
(C) Cystathioninuria
(D) Maple syrup urine disease
(E) Histidinemia

286. The appropriate anticonvulsant therapy for a newborn actively having seizures is

(A) diazepam, 0.3 mg/kg IV
(B) phenytoin, 10 mg/kg IM
(C) rectal paraldehyde
(D) phenobarbital, 20 mg/kg IV
(E) none of the above

287. Diagnosis of which of the following lipidoses is confirmed by the absence of hexosaminidase A activity in white blood cells?

(A) Niemann-Pick disease
(B) Infantile Gaucher's disease
(C) Tay-Sachs disease
(D) Krabbe's disease
(E) Fabry's disease

288. Following a head injury, seizures are most likely to occur in a child within which of the following time periods?

(A) Immediately
(B) Within one week
(C) Within two years
(D) Between two and four years
(E) None of the above time periods

289. In children, the most common type of tumor of the central nervous system is

(A) meningioma
(B) glioma
(C) craniopharyngioma
(D) chordoma
(E) neurinoma

290. A subdural effusion most commonly accompanies meningitis caused by

(A) *Escherichia coli*
(B) *Hemophilus influenzae*
(C) *Neisseria meningitidis*
(D) *Pseudomonas aeruginosa*
(E) *Streptococcus (Diplococcus) pneumoniae*

291. The pictured abnormality may be associated with

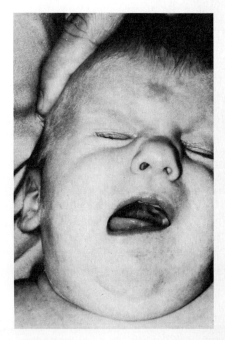

(A) loss of taste
(B) cardiac and renal anomalies
(C) hyperacusis
(D) parotid tumor
(E) ptosis

292. A previously healthy seven-year-old child suddenly complains of a headache and falls to the floor. When examined in the emergency room, he is lethargic and has a left central facial weakness and left hemiparesis with conjugate ocular deviation to the right. The most likely diagnosis is

(A) hemiplegic migraine
(B) supratentorial tumor
(C) Todd's paralysis
(D) acute subdural hematoma
(E) acute infantile hemiplegia

293. A three-year-old child can be expected to do all of the following EXCEPT

(A) undress
(B) copy a square
(C) alternate feet when climbing stairs
(D) name one color
(E) speak in short sentences

294. A seven-month-old infant develops head-nodding spells, which consist of a series of four to six nods a minute. These episodes are characteristic of which of the following disorders?

(A) Petit mal seizures
(B) Psychomotor seizures
(C) Focal motor seizures
(D) Infantile spasms
(E) Multiple tics

295. A six-year-old child has unsteady gait and is irritable. Physical examination reveals a very mild left facial weakness, brisk stretch reflexes in all four extremities, bilateral extensor plantar responses, mild hypertonicity of the left upper and lower extremities, and a somewhat unsteady but nonspecific gait; there is no muscular weakness. The most likely diagnosis is

(A) pontine glioma
(B) cerebellar astrocytoma
(C) right cerebral hemisphere tumor
(D) subacute sclerosing panencephalitis
(E) subacute necrotizing leukoencephalopathy

296. Seizures associated with the pictured EEG segment can be treated with

(A) ethosuximide
(B) carbamazepine
(C) phenytoin
(D) phenobarital
(E) none of the above

297. A ten-year-old child complains of episodic abdominal discomfort; the child's mother says that these episodes are associated with periods of staring and followed by a brief period of lethargy. Which of the following disorders is most likely to be responsible for the child's symptoms?

(A) Pyschomotor seizures
(B) Migraine
(C) Petit mal epilepsy
(D) Conversion reaction
(E) None of the above

298. Which of the following signs or symptoms must be present in a child's history in order to support the diagnosis of concussion following a head injury?

(A) Repeated vomiting
(B) Brief unconsciousness
(C) Drowsiness
(D) Seizure activity
(E) None of the above

299. Brain death implies that there is irreversible injury to such a degree that there is total absence of brainstem function, i.e., no oculocephalic reflex or oculovestibular response, no gag reflex, and no respiratory activity without ventilator support. An isoelectric ("flat") EEG has been used in support of this diagnosis. Which of the following may cause a reversible clinical picture of brain death replete with an isoelectric EEG?

(A) Hyperthermia
(B) Brainstem infarction
(C) Acute alcohol intoxication
(D) Barbiturate intoxication
(E) Reye's syndrome

300. A ten-year-old child who has acute lymphocytic leukemia is lethargic and unsteady. There is no evidence of hematuria or bleeding into the skin. Neurologic examination shows that the child has a mild spastic hemiparesis and hyperreflexia in all extremities; papilledema, however, is not present. Three months ago, the child was treated with 3000 rads of radiation to the head as well as with intrathecal methotrexate for meningeal leukemia.

The child's current neurologic disturbances most likely are the result of

(A) fungal infection
(B) hydrocephalus
(C) meningeal leukemia
(D) leukoencephalopathy
(E) intracerebral hemorrhage

301. Headache, vomiting, and papilledema are common symptoms and signs in children who have brain tumors. Which of the following signs also is frequently associated with craniopharyngioma?

(A) Sixth-nerve palsy
(B) Unilateral cerebellar ataxia
(C) Unilateral pupillary dilatation
(D) Unilateral anosmia
(E) Bitemporal hemianopia

302. The most common location in children for tumors of the nervous system is

(A) subtentorial
(B) supratentorial
(C) intraventricular
(D) in the spinal canal
(E) none of the above

303. Which of the following sets of clinical signs is most likely to be associated with the CAT scan (contrast positive) shown below?

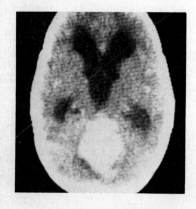

(A) Papilledema, hemparesis, and ipsilateral VIth-nerve and VIIth-nerve palsies
(B) Papilledema, unilateral dysmetria, and falling to the same side
(C) Retinal angiomas, ataxia, and dysmetria
(D) Papilledema and ataxia without dysmetria
(E) None of the above

304. Erb's palsy is described best as

(A) weakness of a wrist and ipsilateral Horner's syndrome
(B) weakness of an arm from a fracture of the head of the humerus
(C) weakness of an arm from a traction injury of the upper brachial plexus
(D) total ipsilateral arm weakness resulting from a fracture of a clavicle
(E) pseudoparalysis of an arm due to syphilitic osteochondritis

305. A newborn infant has marked muscular weakness of the extremities and tongue fasciculations. The mother reports her child was relatively inactive in utero. The most likely diagnosis is

(A) infantile spinal muscular atrophy
(B) Duchenne muscular dystrophy
(C) myotonic dystrophy
(D) myasthenia gravis
(E) fiber type I disproportion

306. The calcific densities in the skull x-ray shown below are likely to have been caused by

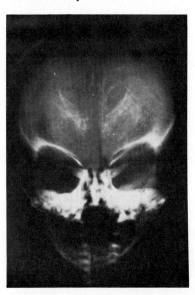

(A) congenital cytomegalovirus infection
(B) congenital toxoplasmosis
(C) congenital syphilis
(D) tuberculous meningitis
(E) craniopharyngioma

307. An infant who has achromic skin patches develops infantile spasms. The disorder most likely to be affecting this infant is

(A) neurofibromatosis
(B) tuberous sclerosis
(C) incontinentia pigmenti
(D) pityriasis rosea
(E) psoriasis

308. The patient whose CAT scan is pictured complained of recurrent headache and vomiting and had papilledema on examination of the fundi. Other features of her disease might include which one of the following conditions?

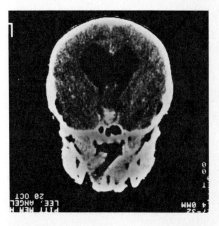

(A) History of a recent head injury
(B) Short stature
(C) Hyperthyroidism
(D) Achromic skin patches
(E) Multiple café au lait lesions

DIRECTIONS: Each question below contains four suggested answers of which **one or more** is correct. Choose the answer:

A	if	**1, 2, and 3**	are correct
B	if	**1 and 3**	are correct
C	if	**2 and 4**	are correct
D	if	**4**	is correct
E	if	**1, 2, 3, and 4**	are correct

309. Symmetrically small pupils in an unconscious patient may be found in

(1) metabolic coma
(2) pontine hemorrhage
(3) heroin-induced coma
(4) atropine-induced coma

310. Congenital defects frequently associated with the radiographic findings illustrated below include

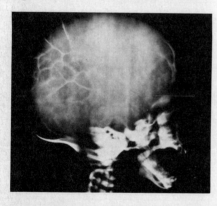

(1) meningomyelocele
(2) cleft lip and palate
(3) encephalocele
(4) craniosynostosis

311. Gowers' maneuver is used by children who have

(1) pseudohypertrophic muscular dystrophy
(2) limb-girdle dystrophy
(3) late-onset spinal muscular atrophy
(4) congenital myopathy

312. A ten-year-old child has pes cavus and scoliosis; other disorders likely to be exhibited by this child include

(1) diminished vibration and position sense
(2) gait and station ataxia
(3) nystagmus
(4) hyperreflexia

313. By three months of age most normal full-term infants can be expected to

(1) move their heads from side to side 180 degrees while following a moving object
(2) lift their heads from a prone position 45 degrees off the examining table
(3) smile when encouraged
(4) maintain a seated position

314. Frontal baldness, cataracts, distal muscle weakness, ptosis, and facial muscle weakness are some of the symptoms of myotonic dystrophy in adults. Children who have this disease commonly exhibit

(1) psychomotor retardation
(2) seizure activity
(3) cardiac arrhythmias
(4) a failure to thrive

315. Clinical characteristics of childhood migraine include

(1) strong family history for migraine
(2) bifrontal headaches
(3) male preponderance before age 12 years
(4) duration of headaches more than 24 hours

316. Intracranial calcifications can appear in infants who have a congenital infection with

(1) *Treponema pallidum*
(2) *Toxoplasma gondii*
(3) rubella virus
(4) cytomegalovirus

317. Intracranial hemorrhage may result from a difficult delivery and from asphyxia or hypoxia. Common sites of bleeding in full-term infants include

(1) intraventricular
(2) posterior fossa
(3) subarachnoid
(4) subdural

318. Examination of the cerebrospinal fluid of an eight-year-old, stuporous, mildly febrile child shows the following: white blood cells, 200/mm^3 (all lymphocytes); protein, 150 mg/100 ml; and glucose, 15 mg/100 ml. Blood glucose concentration is 70 mg/100 ml. The differential diagnosis should include

(1) aseptic meningitis
(2) tuberculous meningitis
(3) meningeal leukemia
(4) medulloblastoma

319. Low cerebrospinal fluid (CSF) sugar is commonly associated with bacterial meningitis, but it may also be found in which of the following disorders?

(1) Hypoglycemia
(2) Subarachnoid hemorrhage
(3) Mumps meningitis
(4) Spinal cord tumor

320. Although valproic acid is widely used as an anticonvulsant, particularly for patients with petit mal seizures, there are side effects, which include

(1) hepatotoxicity
(2) hypotension
(3) interference with other anticonvulsants
(4) drug rash

321. The differential diagnosis for a newborn infant who has multiple joint contractures should include

(1) spinal muscular atrophy
(2) congenital muscular dystrophy
(3) congenital myopathies
(4) myelomeningocele

SUMMARY OF DIRECTIONS

A	B	C	D	E
1,2,3 only	1,3 only	2,4 only	4 only	All are correct

322. No precise definition exists for grand mal status epilepticus. This disorder generally can be defined by which of the following criteria?

(1) One seizure lasting no less than a half hour
(2) Continuous tonic-clonic activity
(3) Repeated seizures with no return to consciousness between them
(4) Several sets of repeated focal seizures occuring in a twenty-four- hour period

323. The calcifications shown on the skull x-ray below can be associated with which of the following?

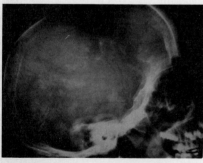

(1) Von Hippel-Lindau disease
(2) Ataxia-telangiectasia
(3) Tuberous sclerosis
(4) Sturge-Weber syndrome

324. A six-year-old child is hospitalized for observation because of a short period of unconsciousness after a fall from a playground swing. Which of the following signs or symptoms would suggest the development of an extradural hematoma?

(1) Unilateral pupillary dilatation
(2) Focal seizures
(3) Recurrence of depressed consciousness
(4) Headache

325. Many diseases of the nervous system are inherited. Of the following, those that are considered to be autosomal dominant include

(1) familial dysautonomia
(2) Huntington chorea
(3) Wilson's disease
(4) neurofibromatosis

326. The differential diagnosis of acute ataxia of childhood should include

(1) drug intoxication
(2) bacterial meningitis
(3) postinfectious viral syndrome
(4) neuroblastoma

327. A newborn infant is noted to have facial diplegia and difficulty sucking and swallowing. Which of the following disorders should be included in the differential diagnosis?

(1) Infantile spinal muscular atrophy
(2) Myasthenia gravis
(3) Myotonic dystrophy
(4) Duchenne muscular dystrophy

328. Bloody cerebrospinal fluid (CSF) produced by a traumatic lumbar puncture can be distinguished from true bloody CSF due to other causes by which of the following methods?

(1) Counting red blood cells in more than one tube
(2) Looking for xanthochromia
(3) Repeating the lumbar puncture at a higher interspace
(4) Observing clotting in the CSF

329. A "cherry red spot" is a well-known finding in Tay-Sachs disease. It may also be found in children with

(1) GM1 type 1 generalized gangliosidosis
(2) GM2 type 2 Sandhoff disease
(3) Niemann-Pick disease, type A
(4) metachromatic leukodystrophy

330. Neonatal seizures can develop as the result of

(1) hypocalcemia
(2) hypoxia
(3) birth trauma
(4) anomalies of the central nervous system

331. True statements about febrile seizures include which of the following?

(1) They usually occur in association with infection of the central nervous system
(2) Most last less than 15 minutes
(3) Affected children usually are between six months and three years of age
(4) Generalized tonic-clonic activity is typical

332. Which of the following are associated with jitteriness in the newborn?

(1) Hypoxic encephalopathy
(2) Hypoglycemia
(3) Drug withdrawal
(4) Hypocalcemia

333. Physical findings characteristic of children who have Sturge-Weber syndrome include

(1) hemiplegia
(2) angiomas of the lips and mouth
(3) a "port wine" nevus on the forehead
(4) an angioma of the retina

334. Laboratory findings consistently associated with Reye's syndrome include which of the following?

(1) Prolonged prothrombin time
(2) Elevated levels of serum transaminases
(3) Elevated blood ammonia levels
(4) Elevated blood glucose levels

335. An asymmetric Moro reflex can be elicited at least occasionally from infants who have

(1) a fractured clavicle
(2) infantile hemiplegia
(3) a brachial plexus palsy
(4) neonatal myasthenia gravis

The Neuromuscular System

Answers

281. The answer is E. *(Shapiro, Semin Neurol 2:375, 1982.)* The clinical characteristics of Tourette syndrome are multiple tics, involving the face, head and neck, shoulders, and limbs, and vocal tics, such as sniffing, snorting, throat clearing, and other vocal tics. This disorder does not have a recognized antecedent illness or CNS insult as its cause in contrast to other movement disorders. There may be a genetic factor, as epidemiologic studies have identified other family members with the same disorder. The drug of choice for treatment is haloperidol. Clonidine has been used as a second choice.

282. The answer is E. *(Bell, vol 12. p 293.)* The infective agent considered to cause subacute sclerosing panencephalitis is measles virus. The presumption is based on the associated central nervous system pathology, which is consistent with encephalitis and features intranuclear and intracytoplasmic inclusion bodies. In addition, measles (rubeola) antibody titers in serum and cerebrospinal fluid are higher than those found in children recovering from measles, a finding that suggests a continuing infective process.

283. The answer is D. *(Volpe, pp 117–118.)* Tonic seizures in the premature infant may actually represent decerebrate/decorticate posturing in association with intraventricular bleeding. Because the latter is commonly a sequela of hypoxic encephalopathy, these episodes may then be brainstem dysfunction rather than cortical events. Apneic spells are a common problem in the premature infant. Those reflecting seizure activity most often are in combination with other activity such as chewing movement or intermittant nystagmus. Breath-holding spells do occur in infancy but not in the newborn period and are of two types, cyanotic and pallid, either of which may conclude with tonic and even brief clonic activity. Maternal drug abuse can cause jitteriness and even seizures in the newborn period. The seizures are usually clonic rather than opisthotonic/tonic.

284. The answer is D. *(Bell, vol 12. pp 272–273.)* Microcephaly, cataracts, congenital heart defects, vasomotor instability, and developmental retardation are among the many disturbances of the congenital rubella syndrome. Deafness, however, is thought to be the single most common defect associated with this disorder. Although the hearing loss seems to involve the inner ear and result primarily in a sensorineural defect, middle-ear damage also has been suggested as an etiologic factor.

285. The answer is B. *(Menkes, ed 2. pp 1–7, 14–16, 21–25.)* Homocystinuria can cause thromboembolic phenomena in the pulmonary and renal arteries and in the cerebral vasculature; vascular occlusive disease is, in turn, one of the many causes of acute infantile hemiplegia. None of the other disorders listed in the question are associated with acute hemiplegia. Phenylketonuria causes retardation and, on occasion, seizures; maple syrup urine disease, an abnormality of the metabolism of leucine, leads to seizures and rapid deterioration of the central nervous system in newborn infants; histidinemia seems to be associated with speech impairments and other minor neurologic difficulties; and cystathioninuria is most likely a benign aminoaciduria having no effect on the central nervous system.

286. The answer is D. *(Bergman, Semin Perinatol 6:54–67, 1982.)* The most appropriate anticonvulsant for the convulsing newborn is intravenous phenobarbital, 20 mg/kg IV. This may be repeated for one to two further doses if seizures are not under control. Phenytoin is the next drug of choice, but it can only be given intravenously. The dosage is 15 to 20 mg/kg. If given intramuscularly, it will crystalize and be poorly absorbed, possibly causing a sterile abscess. Diazepam is effective in controlling major motor status epilepticus in children and adults, but is not recommended in the newborn period. Drugs given per rectum may not achieve adequate serum levels for seizure control.

287. The answer is C. *(Adams and Lyon, pp 43–46, 58–62, 272–274.)* Children who have Tay-Sachs disease are characterized by progressive developmental deterioration; physical signs include macular "cherry red" spots and exquisite sensitivity to noise. Diagnosis of this disorder can be confirmed biochemically by the absence of hexosaminidase A activity in white blood cells. Tay-Sachs disease is inherited as an autosomal recessive trait; about 80 percent of affected children are of eastern European Jewish ancestry. The other disorders listed in the question are associated with enzyme deficiencies as follows: Niemann-Pick disease, sphingomyelinase; infantile Gaucher's disease, β-glucosidase; Krabbe's disease (globoid cell leukodystrophy), galactocerebroside β-galactosidase; and Fabry's disease, α-galactosidase.

288. The answer is B. *(Jennett, ed 2. pp 35–39, 68–69, 91, 93.)* Seizures that result from a head injury fall into two categories: early epilepsy and late epilepsy. The former type occurs within the first week following the injury, while the latter does not appear until three months to as much as ten years later. Children, especially those under five years of age, are more likely to have early epilepsy than are adults, in whom late epilepsy is more common.

289. The answer is B. *(Rudolph, ed 17. pp 1622, 1627,1630.)* Gliomas – for example, astrocytoma, pontine glioma, and optic glioma – comprise 75 percent of intracranial tumors in children and 45 percent in adults. After leukemia, intracranial tumors are the most common type of neoplastic disease among children. Only about 6 percent of brain tumors in children are metastatic.

290. The answer is B. *(Menkes, ed 2. pp 281–282.)* Although subdural effusions can follow all types of acute bacterial meningitis, they most commonly complicate meningitis caused by *Hemophilus influenzae.* How these effusions develop remains uncertain. Abnormal transillumination of the skull as well as certain clinical findings, such as progressive increase in head circumference or occurrence of focal neurologic signs, can suggest the presence of a subdural effusion.

291. The answer is B. *(Nelson, J Pediatr 81:16–20, 1972. Pape, J Pediatr 81:21–30, 1972. Monreal, Pediatrics 65: 146–149, 1980.)* The pictured infant has the so-called asymmetric crying face and not a facial nerve palsy. The former has normal furrowing of the ipsilateral forehead, eye closure, and a normal appearing nasolabial fold during crying. The abnormality results from hypoplasia of the triangularis muscle, the muscle that pulls the corner of the mouth downward and outward. Palpation of the involved side of the lip will reveal diminished bulk compared with the uninvolved side. This anomaly has been associated with others involving the cardiovascular, musculoskeletal, and genitourinary systems.

292. The answer is E. *(Isler, pp 74–102. Menkes, ed 2. pp 264–267.)* The abrupt onset of a hemisyndrome, especially with the eyes looking away from the paralyzed side, strongly indicates a diagnosis of acute infantile hemiplegia. Most frequently this represents a thromboembolic occlusion of the middle cerebral artery or one of its major branches. Hemiplegic migraine commonly occurs in children with a history of migraine headaches. Todd's paralysis follows after a focal or jacksonian seizure and generally does not last more than 24 to 48 hours. The eyes usually look toward the paralyzed side. The clinical onset of a supratentorial brain tumor is subacute with repeated headaches and gradually developing weakness. A history of trauma usually precedes the signs of an acute subdural hematoma. Clinical signs may appear fairly rapidly, but not with the abruptness of occlusive vascular disease.

293. The answer is B. *(Illingworth, ed 7. pp 135, 137, 143, 145, 161.)* Three-year-old children become quite skilled in many areas. Most can say many words and speak in sentences. They are usually toilet trained and can dress and undress themselves with the exception of shoelaces and sometimes buttons. Although they can alternate feet when climbing stairs, they still place both feet on each step when going down stairs. They can identify at least one color by name but have not progressed beyond copying a circle and a crude cross. Only at four to five years of age can a child copy a square.

294. The answer is D. *(Menkes, ed 2. pp 558–560. Singer, J Pediatr 96:485–489, 1980. Hrachovy, J Pediatr 103:641–645, 1983.)* The onset of infantile spasms most commonly occurs in children between the ages of three and eight months. The seizures, which occur in clusters, may take the form of head nodding (with or without arm extension) or spasms of more severe flexion ("salaam seizure"). ACTH (adrenocorticotropin) has been significantly effective in controlling these seizures, though prednisone therapy is thought by some to be equally therapeutic. Normal intellectual development in any infant who has developed infantile spasms is unlikely if there is evidence of prenatal or perinatal neurologic insults, metabolic disorders, or structural abnormalities of the brain. Petit mal, psychomotor seizures, and multiple tics do not occur in infants of this age group. Focal motor seizures may occur at any age but usually involve limbs or facial muscles.

295. The answer is A. *(Altman, pp 314–315.)* A child who has a subacute disorder of the central nervous system producing cranial-nerve abnormalities (especially of the VIIth nerve and the lower bulbar nerves), long-tract signs, unsteady gait secondary to spasticity, and some behavioral changes is most likely to have a pontine glioma. Definitive diagnostic studies would be either pneumoencephalography, which would show enlargement of the pons with posterior displacement of the fourth ventricle, or CAT scan, which also can demonstrate pontine enlargement. Tumors of the cerebellar hemispheres may in later stages produce long-tract signs, but the gait disturbance would be ataxia. Dysmetria and nystagmus also would be present. Supratentorial tumors are quite uncommon in six-year-old children; headache and vomiting would be likely presenting symptoms and papilledema a finding on physical examination.

296. The answer is A. *(Sato, Neurology 32:157–163, 1982.)* The pictured EEG is fairly typical of petit mal absence: generalized 3 c/s spike and slow wave activity. The spells are usually brief, consisting of staring with eye blinking, lack of awareness, and minor motor activity such as chewing or lip smacking. Ethosuximide is effective in most cases. Alternatively, valproic acid can be used with no less effectiveness. The other three medications are used to treat major motor seizures.

297. The answer is A. *(Menkes, ed 2. pp 553–556.)* The consecutive appearance of abdominal distress, staring, and sleepiness or lethargy strongly indicates a paroxysmal disorder. Children who have psychomotor seizures often present in this manner. Other symptoms that have been described include stereotyped motor activity (such as buttoning and unbuttoning of clothes), a sensation of unexplained fearfulness, and déja vu. Affected children may have a history of febrile or grand mal seizures.

298. The answer is B. *(Behrman, ed 12. p 1394.)* Although vomiting and lethargy frequently are associated with a closed head injury, a brief period of unconsciousness always accompanies a concussion. Children old enough to relate their own histories may give evidence of amnesia concerning the events preceding their head injuries (retrograde amnesia) and following their injuries (antegrade amnesia); these historical findings will confirm the diagnosis of concussion. The severity of the injury is generally directly related to the length of time the child was unconscious and the extent of the retrograde amnesia. Children who have had a simple concussion recover fully.

299. The answer is D. *(Rowland, Am J Dis Child 137:547–550, 1983. Black, N Engl J Med 299:338–344. 1978.)* All of the conditions listed in the question can result in coma but need not lead to brain death. To make the diagnosis of brain death, it is necessary to rule out reversible conditions, establish the cause of coma, and treat it if possible. Hypothermia, drug and metabolic intoxications may clinically have the same signs as brain death but indeed are correctable causes of coma in adults as well as children. These agents can produce an EEG of electrocerebral silence ("flat EEG"). On the other hand, brainstem infarction may produce an irreversible coma with total absence of brainstem function but with persistent EEG activity. In some instances, the absence of brainstem auditory evoked potentials, or no flow of radionucleide material into the intracranial circulation will be needed to corroborate the irreversible nature of the coma.

300. The answer is D. *(Neville, Develop Med Child Neurol 14:75–78, 1972. Price, Cancer 35:306–318, 1975. Rubenstein, Cancer 35:291–305, 1975.)* Acute leukemia in children is associated with a number of complications involving the central nervous system. The child described in the question most likely has necrotizing leukoencephalopathy, a recently recognized complication of combined irradiation and intrathecal methotrexate therapy. It has been suggested that irradiation in excess of 2500 rads permits methotrexate to pass into the white matter, resulting in progressive necrosis. Meningeal leukemia, which has become more common with the advent of improved chemotherapy, can lead to hydrocephalus, presumably by infiltration of the arachnoid membrane and consequent obstruction of the flow and absorption of cerebrospinal fluid. Intracerebral hemorrhages usually occur due to thrombocytopenia and produce evidence of bleeding into the skin and other organs. Because of immunosuppression, leukemic children are prone to infection by fungi and yeast.

301. The answer is E. *(Swaiman, ed 2. p 644.)* Upward growth of a craniopharyngioma results in compression of the optic chiasm. Particularly affected are the fibers derived from the nasal portions of both retinas (in other words, from those parts of the eyes receiving stimulation from the temporal visual field). Early in the growth of a craniopharyngioma a unilateral superior quadrantanopic defect can develop; and an irregularly growing tumor can impinge upon the optic chiasm and cause homonymous hemianopia.

302. The answer is A. *(Menkes, ed 2. p 498.)* Between 60 and 70 percent of intracranial tumors in children are located below the tentorium. Of these tumors, the two most common types are medulloblastoma and cerebellar astrocytoma. In adults and infants, most intracranial tumors originate above the tentorium; only 25 to 30 percent of brain tumors in adults are subtentorial.

303. The answer is D. *(Bell, vol 8. pp 359–360, 366–369.)* The CAT scan presented in the question shows dilation of the lateral and third ventricles and a mass filling the fourth ventricle. These findings point to a midline, fourth ventricular tumor, such as a medulloblastoma or ependymoma; clinical signs of these tumors include papilledema and ataxia without dysmetria. The clinical signs of lateralized dysmetria and falling to the same side usually are associated with hemispheric cystic cerebellar astrocytoma; a CAT scan of patients with this disorder can be expected to show a lateralized cystic mass displacing the fourth ventricle to one side. A pontine glioma should be suspected in children who have long-tract signs, either unilaterally or bilaterally, and cranial nerve palsies, especially of the IIId, VIth, and VIIth nerves. Cerebellar hemangioma-blastoma usually occurs in association with a retinal angioma (von Hippel-Lindau syndrome). The clinical signs stemming from bleeding within the tumor depend on the location of the tumor in the cerebellum. Blood can be seen on a CAT scan *without* the use of a contrast agent.

304. The answer is C. *(Menkes, ed 2. pp 269–270.)* Erb's palsy can be caused by traction on an arm during a breech delivery or on the neck during a vertex delivery. Traction results in injury to the upper brachial plexus, causing weakness of the deltoid, biceps, brachialis, and wrist and finger extensor muscles. Recovery is dependent on the degree of nerve injury. Pain caused by osteochondritis of the humerus in an infant who has congenital syphilis (Parrot's pseudoparalysis) inhibits arm movement.

305. The answer is A. *(Brooke, pp 34–36. Dubowitz, p 149.)* Infantile spinal muscular atrophy (Werdnig-Hoffmann disease) is a progressive degenerative disease of anterior horn cells and bulbar motor nuclei. Fasciculations of the tongue can occur in affected infants; however, because tongue fasciculations can accompany crying in normal infants, only the demonstration of fasciculations while a child is at rest will support a diagnosis of infantile spinal muscular atrophy. Some mothers of affected neonates give a history of slowed or arrested fetal movement prior to the onset of labor. Because this disease has an autosomal recessive inheritance pattern, muscle biopsy and examination of histochemically stained specimens should be done to confirm the diagnosis.

306. The answer is A. *(Bell, vol 12. pp 228–236.)* Periventricular calcifications are a characterisitic finding in infants who have congenital cytomegalovirus infection. The encephalitic process especially affects the subependymal tissue around the lateral ventricles and thus results in the periventricular deposition of calcium. Calcified tuberculomas, if visible radiographically, are present around the base of the brain, the preferential site of tuberculous meningitis. Granulomatous encephalitis caused by congenital toxoplasmosis is associated with scattered and soft-appearing intracranial calcification, and suprasellar calcifications are typical of craniopharyngiomas. Congenital syphilis does not produce intracranial calcifications.

307. The answer is B. *(Westmoreland, pp 55–57.)* In infants, achromic skin patches, especially in association with infantile spasms, are pathognomonic for tuberous sclerosis. Other dermal abnormalities (adenoma sebaceum and subungual fibromata) associated with this disorder appear later in childhood. Although children who have neurofibromatosis may have a few achromic patches, the identifying dermal lesions are café au lait spots. Incontinentia pigmenti also is associated with seizures; the skin lesions typical of this disorder begin as bullous eruptions that later become hyperpigmented lesions. Pityriasis rosea and psoriasis are not associated with infantile spasms.

308. The answer is B. *(Thomsett, J Pediatr 97:728–735, 1980.)* The CAT scan of a patient with craniopharyngioma shows hydrocephalus involving the lateral ventricles, a calcific density within the sella, with a mass extending from it compromising the third ventricle. In a recent study of 42 children with craniopharyngioma 43 percent had headache and 35 percent had visual complaints as their initial complaint. Only three were referred for evaluation of delayed growth. However, about one-third of the children were more than two standard deviations below height for their age. Almost all of the children had endocrinologic disturbances of the hypothalamic pituitary axis prior to surgery. Plain skull films can show abnormalities of the sella and/or calcification within or above the sella.

309. The answer is A (1,2,3). *(Plum, ed 3. pp 46–47.)* Pinpoint pupils are found in coma from heroin and pontine hemorrhage. The light reflex is preserved in the former, though it may be difficult to confirm. Small light-reactive pupils are found in metabolic coma, whereas a midbrain injury would produce small, but unresponsive, pupils. Atropine produces dilated pupils, facial flushing, delirium, or stupor.

310. The answer is B (1, 3). *(McRae, Acta Radiol 5:55, 1966.)* Lacunar skull results from abnormal membranous bone formation; it probably begins in utero and resolves by six months of age. The cause is not known but, contrary to popular belief, does not have any relation to increased intracranial pressure, even though it is associated frequently with encephalocele or meningomyelocele. Thinning of bone, which occurs in the thickest parts of the frontal, parietal, and upper portion of the occipital bones, creates the impression that there are holes in the skull.

311. The answer is E (all). *(Brooke, p 41. Dubowitz, pp 24–26.)* Gowers' maneuver is characteristic of individuals who have proximal muscle weakness of the pelvic girdle, regardless of the etiology. These individuals, when wishing to arise after lying down, must become prone and gradually stand by using their hands to "walk" up their legs. Not specific just for Duchenne (pseudohypertrophic) muscular dystrophy, Gowers' maneuver also is used by children who have limb-girdle dystrophy, late-onset spinal muscular dystrophy, and congenital myopathy.

312. The answer is A (1, 2, 3). *(Menkes, ed 2. pp 118–122.)* Friedreich's ataxia, a spinocerebellar degenerative disease, is characterized by both cerebellar and posterior column dysfunction. Pes cavus (high arch) and scoliosis are skeletal hallmarks of this disorder, which can be inherited as either an autosomal dominant or an autosomal recessive trait. Neurologic symptoms frequently encountered include abnormal speech, diminished position and vibration sense, nystagmus, hyporeflexia, and gait and station ataxia. There is no curative treatment for children who have Friedreich's ataxia.

313. The answer is A (1, 2, 3). *(Illingworth, ed 7. pp 133, 140.)* Infants who are developing normally should be able to smile when smiled at or talked to by eight weeks of age. By three months of age, infants should be able to follow a moving toy not only from side to side but also in the vertical plane. When placed on their abdomens, normal three-month-old infants can raise their faces 45 to 90 degrees from the horizontal. Not until infants reach six to eight months of age should they be able to maintain a seated position.

314. The answer is B (1, 3). *(Harper, pp 170–185.)* Psychomotor retardation may be the presenting complaint of children who have myotonic dystrophy. Ptosis, facial immobility, and neonatal respiratory distress are major features of this disorder in the newborn period. Not infrequently the mother may have the disease in a mild form, and a careful family history and examination of the parents, particularly the mother, may be necessary to elicit the diagnosis in an affected infant. Seizures and failure to thrive are not prominent features of myotonic dystrophy.

315. The answer is A (1,2,3). *(Brown, Develop Med Child Neurol 19:683–692, 1977. Prensky, Neurology 29:506–510, 1979.)* In contrast to adults, children with migraine most often have "common" migraine: bifrontal headache without an aura or diffuse throbbing headache of only a few hours duration. Like adults, the headaches may be terminated with vomiting or sleep. Migraine may begin as early as two to three years of age, with boys being affected somewhat more than girls until preteen or early teen years when girls, like adult young women, are more likely to have migraine.

316. The answer is C (2, 4). *(Menkes, ed 2. pp 307, 309.)* Neonates who have congenital syphilis, rubella, toxoplasmosis, or cytomegalic inclusion disease all have jaundice and hepatosplenomegaly. Only the latter two diseases, however, are associated with intracranial calcification. In infants who have congenital toxoplasmosis, intracranial calcifications occur in scattered locations in the brain. Calcium deposits in infants who have a cytomegaloviral infection, on the other hand, appear in subependymal tissue; as a consequence, these calcifications tend to outline the ventricular system.

317. The answer is C (2, 4). *(Volpe, pp 762–769.)* Intraventricular or germinal matrix hemorrhage with rupture into the lateral ventricle is most commonly seen in hypoxic premature infants. Hypoxia and prematurity are also the common predisposing factors for subarachnoid hemorrhage. In contrast, subdural and posterior fossa hemorrhages are sequelae of difficult deliveries with torsion and tearing of major venous channels. Subdural hemorrhages result from rupture of superficial veins, and posterior fossa hemorrhages from tears of tentorial veins or veins of Galen.

318. The answer is E (all). *(Bell, vol 12. pp 79–80.)* Aseptic meningitis, tuberculous meningitis, meningeal leukemia, and medulloblastoma all can cause pleocytosis as well as elevated protein and lowered glucose concentrations in cerebrospinal fluid. Of the four diseases, tuberculous meningitis is associated with the lowest cerebrospinal fluid glucose levels. The cellular response to viral (aseptic) meningitis will be predominantly lymphocytic. Cells found in the cerebrospinal fluid of a child who has meningeal leukemia most commonly are lymphocytes or lymphoblasts. Children who have a medulloblastoma generally present with the signs and symptoms caused by a mass in the posterior cranial fossa; their pleocytotic cerebrospinal fluid contains unusual-appearing cells of the monocytic variety. The decrease in the cerebrospinal glucose concentration associated with these disorders has been attributed to a disturbance of glucose transport as a result of meningeal irritation.

319. The answer is E (all). *(Fishman, pp 208–214.)* Low cerebrospinal fluid (CSF) sugar (hypoglycorrachia) is found in all of the conditions listed in the question. The amount of glucose in CSF reflects both entry and exit of the glucose in and out of the CSF space as well as its utilization by cellular elements bordering that space. The CSF sugar level tends to be 60 to 80 percent of that in the plasma; therefore, hypoglycorrachia is found in conjunction with hypoglycemia. In bacterial infections of the central nervous system, such as mumps meningitis, low CSF sugar results from increased utilization by the adjacent arachnoid, ependyma, glia, and neurones and, in small part, by the polymorphonuclear leukocytes and impaired transmembranal transport. This also may hold true for subarachnoid hemorrhage, but it does not account for the low CSF sugar below the block caused by a malignant tumor, the cause of which remains unknown.

320. The answer is B (1, 3). *(Browne, N Engl J Med 302:661–665, 1980.)* There have been several reported deaths believed due to liver failure in patients being treated with valproic acid. It is necessary to measure a patient's serum aspartate aminotransferase (serum glutamic-oxaloacetic transaminase, SGOT) and alanine aminotransferase (serum glutamic-pyruvic transaminase, SGPT) on a monthly basis when introducing the drug, and at three- to six-month intervals when the maintenance dosage has been achieved. If elevation of these enzymes occurs, they may respond to reduction of dosage; however, if they exceed three times the upper limit of normal or are associated with other indications of altered liver function, the medication should be discontinued. While valproic acid may increase the serum level of phenobarbital and cause signs of toxicity, it also may decrease the total phenytoin level without increasing the free (active) serum phenytoin. This could result in increased seizure activity.

321. The answer is E (all). *(Dubowitz, pp 232–235. Walton, ed 4. pp 645–646.)* Multiple joint contractures in newborn infants are symptoms of diseases of muscle or of disturbances in muscle innervation. The clinical picture associated with these contractures has been called arthrogryposis multiplex congenita. Infants who have a myelomeningocele frequently have contractures of ankle and knee joints as a result of the spinal cord defect and immobilization of the lower extremities in utero.

322. The answer is A (1, 2, 3). *(Delgado-Escueta, pp 3–14.)* Although no exact definition of grand mal status epilepticus now exists, there is general agreement that the term implies either repeated seizures without a lucid, responsive interval or a grand mal seizure lasting at least a half hour. Some neurologists prefer to use the criterion of continuous tonic-clonic activity for one hour. Grand mal status epilepticus occurs more commonly than petit mal or psychomotor status and, if not treated, is the most serious and potentially lethal of the three. It can develop secondarily to a central nervous system infection, a toxic metabolic state, or a primary seizure disorder.

323. The answer is D (4). *(Caffey, ed 7. p 239.)* The parallel linear calcifications ("tram line" calcifications) seen in the skull x-ray presented in the question are typical of Sturge-Weber syndrome. These calcifications lie within the cerebral cortex; they are not associated with the intracranial vascular malformations common in individuals who have this syndrome. Sturge-Weber syndrome is an inherited disorder associated with a high incidence of mental retardation.

324. The answer is B (1, 3). *(Menkes, ed 2. pp 421–424.)* Compression of the IIId cranial nerve and distortion of the brainstem, resulting in unilateral pupillary dilatation and depressed consciousness, suggest a progressively enlarging mass, most likely an extradural hematoma. Such a hematoma displaces the temporal lobe into the tentorial notch and presses on the ipsilateral IIId cranial nerve. Pupillary dilatation occurs before IIId cranial nerve pareses. Brainstem compression by this additional tissue mass leads to progressive deterioration in consciousness. A CAT scan is the best method to differentiate this problem from an intracerebral hematoma or focal brain swelling. Seizures are not a frequent complication of head injury in children. Headache following a head injury is a common and nonspecific symptom.

325. The answer is C (2,4). *(Swaiman, ed 2. pp 336–339.)* Huntington chorea and neurofibromatosis share only their inheritance pattern, that of an autosomal dominant disorder. Familial dysautonomia (Riley-Day syndrome) and Wilson's disease (hepatolenticular degeneration) are autosomal recessive diseases. It is important to be aware of the genetic nature of various neurologic disorders in order to provide accurate genetic counseling.

326. The answer is E (all). *(Bell, vol 12. pp 434–436.)* Cerebellar ataxia in childhood most commonly occurs in association with a mild viral syndrome or viral exanthem. Ingestion – whether intentional or accidental – of barbiturates, phenytoin, or alcohol also must be considered. Children who have bacterial meningitis can present, though rarely, with acute ataxia. Ataxia, opsoclonus (chaotic eye movements), and myoclonus comprise infantile polymyoclonia, which can occur in association with neuroblastoma.

327.   The answer is A (1, 2, 3). *(Brooke, pp 34–36, 131. Dubowitz, pp 139–142, 149, 192–193.)* Spinal muscular atrophy occurring in a neonate is associated with hypotonia and feeding difficulties; a muscle biopsy can confirm this diagnosis. Neonatal myasthenia gravis, though uncommon, must be considered in a newborn infant who has the symptoms described in the question. The symptoms presented also could represent myotonic dystrophy; this diagnosis is confirmed by examination of both parents for percussion and grip myotonia and by electromyographic depiction of myotonic discharges. Duchenne (pseudohypertrophic) muscular dystrophy clinically appears in children who are about two or three years of age.

328.   The answer is A (1, 2, 3). *(Fishman, pp 171–182.)* When bloody cerebrospinal fluid (CSF) results from a subarachnoid hemorrhage, there will be the same number of red blood cells per mm^3 in the first tube as in the third tube of CSF. With a traumatic lumbar puncture there will be more red blood cells in either the first or the third tube with significantly fewer in all the other tubes. A lumbar puncture in a higher interspace repeated immediately will be free of blood if the first puncture was traumatic. The supernatant of traumatically bloody CSF will be clear, while that from a CSF with subarachnoid hemorrhage will demonstrate xanthochromia, usually within two to four hours after the bleeding episode. Because bloody CSF, regardless of cause, rarely clots, observation for clotting will be of no assistance in differentiating the cause.

329.   The answer is A (1,2,3). *(Menkes, ed 2. pp 55–71.)* The cherry red spot represents the center of a normal retinal macula that is surrounded by ganglion cells in which there is an abnormal accumulation of lipid. This alters the surrounding retinal color so that it is yellowish or grayish white. In the first three disorders noted, there is lipid material in the ganglion cells. Metachromatic leukodystrophy does not affect the retina as it is a demyelinating disorder rather than a "storage" disease.

330.   The answer is E (all). *(Volpe, pp 119–124.)* The most frequent causes of neonatal seizures are tetany and birth trauma associated with anoxia. It is not clear in the case of hypocalcemia-related seizures whether the metabolic abnormality acts alone or in addition to brain injury caused by hypoxia to lower the threshold for seizure activity. Anomalies such as proencephaly and agenesis of the corpus callosum may be found in neonates who are having seizures.

331.   The answer is C (2, 4). *(Faerø, Epilepsia 13:279–285, 1972. Nelson, N Engl J Med 295: 1029–1033, 1976.)* Febrile seizures generally occur in children between the ages of six months and three years and usually in association with upper respiratory illness, roseola, shigellosis, or gastroenteritis. The generalized seizures are mostly brief (two to five minutes) and the cerebrospinal fluid is normal. Infants who have seizures that are prolonged (longer than 15 minutes), focal, or lateralized or who had neurologic problems before the febrile seizure are at a higher risk than other affected infants for developing an afebrile seizure disorder during the next five to seven years. These children should be treated on a chronic basis with phenobarbital; blood levels of this drug should be maintained within the therapeutic range of 20 to 40 μ/ml.

332. The answer is E (all). *(Volpe, p 119.)* Jitteriness or rhythmic tremor induced by the stimulation of handling an infant is found in all of the listed circumstances. This motor activity can be distinguished from seizures because it is suppressible by flexing the extremity or merely firmly holding it. In addition, in contrast to seizures, this tremulousness is unaccompanied by apnea, eye deviation, or staring. All of the circumstances listed may also result in neonatal seizures.

333. The answer is A (1, 2, 3). *(Caffey, ed 7. pp 239–240. Swaiman, ed 2. p 790.)* Children who have Sturge-Weber syndrome characteristically can be recognized by the port wine vascular nevus occurring in the distribution of the ophthalmic and maxillary branches of the trigeminal nerve. Angiomas involving the nose, mouth, and lips are not uncommon in these children. Hemiplegia, if present, occurs contralaterally to the port wine stain and leptomeningeal angiomas. Angiomas of the retina, along with cerebellar and spinal cord hemangioblastomas and renal cysts, are characteristic of von Hippel-Lindau disease.

334. The answer is A (1, 2, 3). *(DeVivo, Pediatr Clin North Am 23:527–540, 1976. Pollack, pp 3–14.)* Reye's syndrome should be suspected when a child begins to vomit unremittingly and appears confused, disoriented, or markedly lethargic. This syndrome generally occurs as a child is recovering from a mild viral illness or on the third to fifth day of a chickenpox infection. Tachypnea and seizures may develop even in the early stages of the disorder. The most characteristic laboratory findings are serum transaminase levels at least two times normal, elevated levels of blood ammonia, and prothrombin times that are two or more seconds longer than in controls. Hypoglycemia also is common, particularly in younger children. Specific treatment remains controversial, but good supportive care and management of brain edema and increased intracranial pressure are essential.

335. The answer is A (1, 2, 3). *(Gordon, p 6.)* The most common causes of an asymmetric Moro reflex in infants are injuries to the brachial plexus and clavicular fractures. Humeral, radial, and ulnar fractures also may produce an asymmetric response. Infantile hemiplegia, too, is associated, though less commonly than the factors listed above, with an asymmetric Moro reflex.

Infectious Diseases and Immunology

Cody Meissner

DIRECTIONS: Each question below contains five suggested answers. Choose the **one best** response to each question.

336. Which of the following viruses has not been associated with congenital infections?

(A) Cytomegalovirus
(B) Rubella virus
(C) Hepatitis B virus
(D) Herpes simplex virus
(E) Rotavirus

337. A 15-year-old boy develops fever and tachypnea following five days of sore throat, headache, and gradually worsening cough. Chest x-ray shows bilateral hilar infiltrates. White blood cell count is normal. Gram stain of a nasopharyngeal swab shows large numbers of lancet-shaped gram-positive diplococci. The causative organism most likely is

(A) *Streptococcus (Diplococcus) pneumoniae*
(B) *Mycoplasma pneumoniae*
(C) *Mycoplasma hominis*
(D) *Mycobacterium tuberculosis*
(E) *Legionella pneumophila*

338. Following a mild two-week upper respiratory tract infection, a six-month-old girl develops a severe cough that is not relieved by expectorants. The cough is paroxysmal and exhausting, and copious amounts of sticky, clear mucus issue from the nose and mouth. Treatment with ampicillin is ineffective, and hospitalization is required after a brief convulsion during a coughing spell on the tenth day following onset of the severe cough.

A presumptive diagnosis of this child's disorder can be made by a

(A) throat culture
(B) white blood cell count
(C) chest x-ray
(D) Gram stain of the tracheal aspirate
(E) Gram stain of the nasal discharge

339. All of the following are recognized complications of chickenpox EXCEPT

(A) Reye's syndrome
(B) encephalitis
(C) pneumonia
(D) hemorrhagic varicella
(E) orchitis

340. The best single-drug treatment for individuals who have meningitis caused by *Hemophilus influenzae*, type B, is with intravenous

(A) ampicillin
(B) gentamicin
(C) cephalothin
(D) chloramphenicol
(E) erythromycin

341. An eight-year-old boy who has no history of sexual contact develops dysuria and a purulent urethral discharge. Culture on chocolate agar shows a few colonies of *Escherichia coli*. Forty-eight hours later, his left ankle becomes swollen, hot, and tender, coincident with the onset of chills, fever, and a stiff neck. A lumbar puncture shows cloudy cerebrospinal fluid. The cause of this disease is most likely to be

(A) *Neisseria gonorrhoeae*
(B) *Mycoplasma hominis*
(C) T-strain *Mycoplasma*
(D) *Chlamydia*
(E) herpesvirus hominis, type 2

342. A 14-year-old boy is seen in the emergency room because of a three-week history of fever between 101° and 102°F, lethargy, and a 6-lb. weight loss. Physical examination reveals marked cervical and inguinal adenopathy, enlarged tonsils with exudate, and a palpable spleen 2 cm below the left costal margin. The pediatrician suspects infectious mononucleosis. All of the following conditions would be consistent with that diagnosis EXCEPT

(A) small hemorrhages on the soft palate
(B) a WBC differential revealing 50 percent lymphocytes and 10 percent atypical lymphocytes
(C) a positive heterophil titer
(D) antibodies to EBV viral capsid antigen at a titer of 1:512
(E) a vesicular exanthem

343. All of the following statements about acute osteomyelitis are true EXCEPT that

(A) it most commonly is caused by *Staphylococcus aureus*
(B) it often arises following development of deep cellulitis
(C) tenderness in the region of infection is diffuse, not localized
(D) bony changes are not visible radiographically for five to ten days after onset of infection
(E) antibiotic therapy usually is required for at least four weeks

344. A three-year-old boy has had a temperature of 39°C (102.2°F) and a stiff back for the last three days. Examination shows a red throat, large non-tender anterior and posterior cervical nodes, and slight resistance of the neck to flexion. Immediate management should include a

(A) lumbar puncture
(B) heterophil test
(C) throat culture and oral penicillin for seven days
(D) throat culture and oral penicillin for ten days
(E) throat culture, white blood cell count, and reexamination in 24 hours

345. An eight-day old infant male with staphylococcal pneumonia is at risk for all of the following complications EXCEPT

(A) pneumatocele formation
(B) pneumothorax
(C) empyema
(D) pleural effusion
(E) epiglottitis

346. A 14-month-old infant suddenly develops a fever of 40.2°C (104.4°F). Physical examination shows an alert, active infant who drinks milk eagerly. No physical abnormalities are noted. The white blood cell count is 22,000/mm^3 with 78 percent polymorphonuclear leukocytes, 18 percent of which are band forms. The most likely diagnosis is

(A) pneumococcal bacteremia
(B) roseola
(C) streptococcosis
(D) typhoid fever
(E) diphtheria

347. The leading cause of bacterial meningitis in children between the ages of six months and three years

(A) group A β-hemolytic streptococci
(B) group C *Neisseria meningitidis*
(C) type 5 *Streptococcus (Diplococcus) pneumoniae*
(D) type b *Hemophilus influenzae*
(E) untypable *Hemophilus influenzae*

348. A three-year-old child awakens at night with a fever of 39.6°C (103.3°F), a severe sore throat, and a barking cough. Physical examination of the child, who is drooling, shows a very red throat and inspiratory stridor. The hypopharynx is obscured by yellow mucus. The lungs are clear and there is no respiratory distress. Optimal management would include

(A) immediate hospitalization for possible intubation
(B) immediate inhalation therapy with racemic epinephrine
(C) treatment with oral ampicillin, 50 mg/kg per day
(D) suctioning of the pharynx and hourly examinations of the hypopharynx
(E) a throat culture and initiation of expectorant and mist therapy

349. A three-day-old infant develops *Escherichia coli* meningitis. Treatment with intravenous chloramphenicol, 40 mg/kg daily, produces prompt clinical improvement; beginning on the fifth day of therapy, however, she becomes progressively lethargic and refuses feedings. Because her temperature is subnormal, she is placed on a heated bed. No specific physical or hematologic abnormalities are found, and examination of cerebrospinal fluid shows improvement over results obtained five days earlier.

For the immediate management of this child, the physician involved should

(A) obtain an electroencephalogram
(B) obtain a CAT scan of the skull
(C) begin a treatment with ampicillin
(D) increase the dose of chloramphenicol
(E) reduce the dose of chloramphenicol

350. Which of the following infections typically has an incubation period of less than two weeks?

(A) Mumps
(B) Varicella
(C) Rubella
(D) Measles
(E) Rabies

351. A 14-year-old girl awakens with a mild sore throat, low-grade fever, and a diffuse maculopapular rash. During the next 24 hours she develops tender swelling of her wrists and redness of her eyes. In addition, her physician notes mild tenderness and marked swelling of her posterior cervical and occipital lymph nodes. Four days after the onset of her illness the rash has vanished.

The most likely diagnosis of this girl's condition is

(A) rubella
(B) rubeola
(C) roseola
(D) erythema infectiosum
(E) erythema multiforme

352. Which of the following statements about measles encephalitis is true?

(A) It occurs relatively rarely (1 per 10,000 cases of measles)
(B) It occurs more frequently in association with severe rather than mild cases of measles
(C) An immunologic demyelinating reaction may play a role in development of the disease
(D) It is not associated with the vaccine strain of virus
(E) The prognosis usually depends on the degree of coma

353. The management of salmonellal gastroenteritis ordinarily includes the administration of

(A) ampicillin
(B) chloramphenicol
(C) tetracycline
(D) cephaloridine
(E) none of the above

354. A five-year-old boy develops a mild sore throat, malaise, a low-grade fever, and a faint, generalized, rough, fine red papular rash most obvious on the trunk. His tongue is coated as shown in figure A below. After three days the rash has faded, and his tongue appears as in figure B. One week later there is a sudden, alarming loss of the superficial layers of skin from his fingers.

The most likely diagnosis of this child's condition is

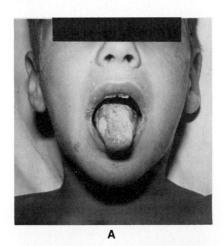

A

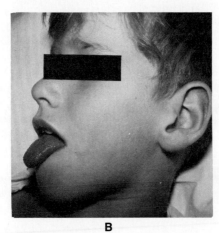

B

(A) rubella
(B) fifth disease
(C) roseola
(D) scarlet fever
(E) thrush

355. Rocky Mountain spotted fever is an acute illness characterized by fever, muscle pain, and a rash that is most prominent on the extremities. The disease is caused by *Rickettsia rickettsii,* which is transmitted by the bite of a tick. Which of the following might NOT be found in a patient with this diagnosis?

(A) A history of a tick bite nine days prior to presentation
(B) A maculopapular rash that began on the flexor surfaces of the wrist
(C) Evolution of the rash to a hemorrhagic appearance
(D) A low serum sodium associated with thrombocytopenia
(E) A purulent tonsilitis

356. Rocky Mountain spotted fever must always be considered when a child from an endemic area presents with fever and a rash on the extremities. Other possibilities that should be considered in the differential diagnosis of Rocky Mountain spotted fever include all of the following EXCEPT

(A) a petechial rash due to *Neisseria meningitidis*
(B) viral infections
(C) atypical measles
(D) toxic shock syndrome
(E) varicella

357. The rash and mucous-membrane lesions shown below develop in an infant five days after a nonspecific upper respiratory tract infection. Which of the following is LEAST likely to be responsible?

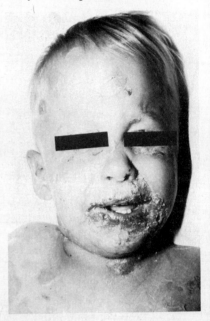

(A) *Mycoplasma pneumoniae*
(B) Herpesvirus hominis, type 1
(C) Rubella virus
(D) Phenobarbital ingestion
(E) Penicillin therapy

358. Which of the following statements about aplastic anemia caused by chloramphenicol therapy is correct?

(A) It occurs with an incidence of about 0.01 percent
(B) It is usually dose-related
(C) It disappears when treatment is discontinued
(D) It appears during therapy rather than after therapy
(E) None of the above

359. A 15-year-old boy develops the acute onset of abdominal pain, watery diarrhea, and nausea ten hours after eating in his favorite Oriental restaurant. The most likely cause of his diarrhea is which of the following?

(A) *Bacillus cereus*
(B) *Campylobacter jejuni*
(C) *Salmonella*
(D) *Escherichia coli*
(E) *Yersinia enterocolitica*

360. Streptococcal pyoderma (impetigo) is best described as

(A) a vesicular or bullous infection in which the blisters rupture over a period of many hours
(B) a vesicular infection in which blisters rupture early and crusts develop
(C) a vesicular infection characterized by painful brown, crusted lesions that spread out on the face
(D) a vesicular infection producing painful, indurated, thick-walled vesicles on a red fingertip
(E) a vesicular infection in which painful vesicles are arranged in a linear pattern

DIRECTIONS: Each question below contains four suggested answers of which **one or more** is correct. Choose the answer:

A	if	**1, 2, and 3**	are correct
B	if	**1 and 3**	are correct
C	if	**2 and 4**	are correct
D	if	**4**	is correct
E	if	**1, 2, 3, and 4**	are correct

361. Which of the following statements regarding infant botulism are NOT true?

(1) In infant botulism, the preformed toxin is contained in food ingested by the infant
(2) A distinct prodrome consisting of constipation, poor feeding, weak cry, and loss of head control is often seen
(3) Most infants never show a complete resolution of symptoms
(4) Findings on physical examination include diffuse hypotenia, weak suck, and absent deep tendon reflexes

362. A lumbar puncture of a child who has signs of meningitis shows a white blood cell count of $600/mm^3$ (62% polymorphonuclear leukocytes and 38% lymphocytes) and a glucose level of 40 mg/100 ml (blood glucose is 110 mg/100 ml). Gram staining is unproductive. Organisms likely to cause this clinical picture include

(1) *Mycobacterium tuberculosis*
(2) group A coxsackievirus
(3) *Cryptococcus neoformans*
(4) lymphocytic choriomeningitis virus

363. Twelve hours after eating her Christmas dinner, a three-year-old girl develops vomiting, abdominal cramps, low-grade fever, and profuse watery diarrhea that fails to improve with a clear liquid diet. Stool cultures obtained on the fourth day because of persistent diarrhea show neither *Salmonella* nor *Shigella* species. However, additional studies might be expected to show

(1) *Yersinia enterocolitica*
(2) a rotavirus infection
(3) *Campylobacter fetus*
(4) *Clostridium difficile*

364. A newborn infant has an abnormally small head; skull x-ray is shown below. The radiographic findings are characteristic of infection with which of the following organisms?

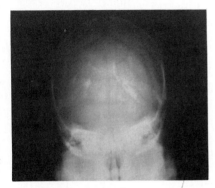

(1) *Toxoplasma gondii*
(2) *Treponema pallidum*
(3) Cytomegalovirus
(4) Rubella virus

365. Infectious mononucleosis is primarily a disease caused by the Epstein-Barr virus (EBV). A patient with this disease usually has a triad of findings consisting of the appropriate changes in physical exam, the associated serologic changes, and the corresponding hematologic abnormalities. Which of the following statements about infectious mononucleosis are true?

(1) The incubation period is four to six weeks
(2) Fifteen percent of seropositive individuals excrete virus at any one point
(3) Transmission of the disease is mainly via EBV containing saliva; thus, epidemics do not occur
(4) A person may be infected by an exogenous strain of EBV on more than one occasion

366. A 15-year-old boy returned to his pediatrician because of a persistent, but moderately improved, urethral discharge two weeks following treatment with intramuscular procaine penicillin G, 4.8 million units, and oral probenecid, 1 g. A Gram stain of the original discharge had shown many gram-negative diplococci within abundant leukocytes. When reexamined, no organisms could be identified either by stain or bacteriologic culture. Manifestations of disease in other individuals infected with the boy's persistent pathogen or with related serotypes would be likely to include

(1) persistent tachypnea, cough, and inspiratory rales in a two-month-old infant
(2) purulent conjunctival discharge in a three-day-old infant
(3) fever and tender swollen inguinal lymph nodes
(4) interstitial pneumonia in a sixteen-year-old girl who works in a pet store

367. A newborn infant becomes markedly jaundiced on the second day of life, and a faint petechial eruption first noted at birth is now a generalized purpuric rash. Hematologic studies for hemolytic diseases are negative. Appropriate measures at this time would include

(1) radiographic examination of the long bones
(2) isolation of the infant from pregnant hospital personnel
(3) a blood culture
(4) measurement of the level of serum immunoglobulin M

SUMMARY OF DIRECTIONS

A	B	C	D	E
1,2,3 only	1,3 only	2,4 only	4 only	All are correct

368. Common features of infections with hepatitis A virus include which of the following?

(1) Prolonged presence of virus in stools
(2) Short incubation period (15 to 50 days)
(3) Frequent occurrence of extrahepatic manifestations
(4) Sudden onset of fever, nausea, and vomiting

369. It has been estimated that during the period 1977–1978 there were between five and ten million deaths worldwide due to acute infectious diarrhea. The precise role played by viral gastroenteritis is not clear, although it is safe to state that rotaviruses and the Norwalk-like viruses play an important role. Which of the following statements about rotaviruses is/are NOT true?

(1) The name of the virus is derived from the Latin word rota, which means "wheel," because in the electron microscope the virus particle resembles the rim of a wheel connected by short spokes
(2) Rotavirus is the major pathogen in infantile gastroenteritis
(3) Rotaviral diarrhea is characterized by watery stools with fever and vomiting and isotonic dehydration
(4) Adults are not infected by rotavirus

370. Neurologic complications can develop from the administration of which of the following vaccines?

(1) Oral polio vaccine (Sabin)
(2) Diphtheria-pertussis-tetanus vaccine
(3) Smallpox vaccine
(4) Measles vaccine

371. The standard serologic test for diagnosing mononucleosis induced by Epstein-Barr virus has been the heterophil test. This test is now being supplemented by specific assays that measure antibodies against the Epstein-Barr virus itself. Which of the following statements are true?

(1) In as many as 5 to 10 percent of patients, the heterophil may remain positive for 18 months or longer
(2) The differential heterophil absorption test will not identify patients with serum sickness-like syndrome
(3) Once infected by the Epstein-Barr virus, antibodies against the viral capsid antigen will be present for the life of the host
(4) Not all patients with a primary Epstein-Barr virus infection will have a rise in IgM antibodies to the viral capsid antigen

372. A two-month-old infant has a temperature of 39.6°C (103.3°F); physical examination is completely normal. This child could have which of the following types of infection?

(1) Roseola infantum
(2) Bacterial meningitis
(3) Streptococcal pharyngitis
(4) Urinary tract infection

373. In addition to the familiar maculopapular rash, measles typically is characterized by which of the following symptoms?

(1) Cough
(2) Moderate or high fever
(3) Coryza
(4) Conjunctivitis

374. Correct statements about disease caused by *Candida albicans* include which of the following?

(1) *Candida albicans* may be found in the intestinal tract and on the mucous membranes of normal individuals as a yeast form
(2) Systemic disease caused by *Candida* occurs primarily in individuals who are immunocompromised, have diabetes mellitus, or have received antibiotics and corticosteroids
(3) Chronic mucocutaneous candidiasis is a syndrome associated with defects in T-cell immunity
(4) There is no effective therapy for disseminated disease caused by *Candida*

375. A positive Mantoux test in a child is likely to

(1) develop within two to ten weeks after infection
(2) indicate infection with atypical mycobacteria
(3) indicate a need for antimicrobial therapy
(4) become negative for a brief period after immunization with live viruses

376. A three-year-old black male developed a painful tender swelling of his foot, accompanied by a temperature of 39°C (102.2°F). His white blood cell count was 10,600/mm³ (72% polymorphonuclear leukocytes and 18% lymphocytes), and his erythrocyte sedimentation rate was 56 mm per hour. An x-ray of his foot is shown below. True statements about this child's illness include which of the following?

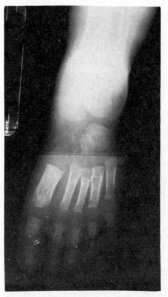

Courtesy of Donald Darling, M.D.

(1) *Salmonella* organisms may be found in his blood
(2) His sodium metabisulfite blood test is likely to be abnormal
(3) Polyvalent pneumococcal vaccine may significantly reduce his future morbidity
(4) Intravenous sodium oxacillin is the treatment of choice

=======================================
SUMMARY OF DIRECTIONS

A	B	C	D	E
1,2,3	**1,3**	**2,4**	**4**	**All are**
only	**only**	**only**	**only**	**correct**
=======================================

377. A ten-year-old boy from the Connecticut coast is seen by his pediatrician because of discomfort in his right knee. A careful history reveals a large annular erythematous lesion on his back that disappeared four weeks prior to the present visit. His mother recalls pulling a tick off his back. Which of the following statements about this child's likely illness are correct?

(1) Lyme disease is an inflammatory process that generally begins with a skin lesion called erythema chronicum migrans
(2) The disease is caused by a spirochete which is transmitted by the bite of a tick
(3) In addition to skin and joint involvement, CNS and cardiac abnormalities may be present
(4) Penicillin therapy results in a more rapid resolution of symptoms than in untreated patients

378. True statements about poliomyelitis include which of the following?

(1) It can be asymptomatic or non-paralytic
(2) It is accompanied by fever, sore throat, and myalgia
(3) Aseptic meningitis can be a prominent feature
(4) Hypertension and urinary retention sometimes arise as complications

379. Meningococcemia can lead to which of the following complications?

(1) Acute adrenal failure
(2) Arthritis
(3) Gastrointestinal hemorrhage
(4) Pericarditis

380. Three days after swellings first appeared at the angle of his mandible, a seven-year-old boy suddenly develops a severe headache, fever, and stiff neck. His cerebrospinal fluid contains 300 leukocytes/mm^3 (62% polymorphonuclear leukocytes and 38% lymphocytes), 40 mg/100 ml of protein, and 60 mg/100 ml of glucose. His blood glucose level is 120 mg/100 ml. His physician should

(1) repeat the lumbar puncture in four to six hours
(2) obtain a serum amylase level
(3) order a heterophil test
(4) begin antibiotic therapy immediately

381. Disease is produced by which of the following parasites in the course of their migration through the parenchyma of body tissues?

(1) *Necator americanus*
(2) *Ascaris lumbricoides*
(3) *Toxocara canis*
(4) *Enterobius vermicularis*

382. A newborn infant has the desquamating rash depicted in the figure below. The child might also be expected to develop which of the following conditions?

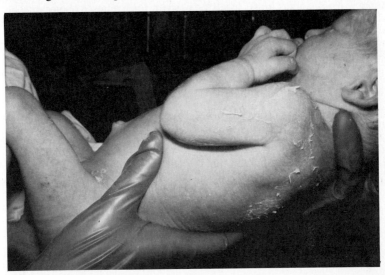

(1) Purulent umbilical drainage
(2) Pneumonia
(3) Progressive enlargement of one breast
(4) An asymmetric Moro reflex

383. A child who has croup can be expected to

(1) have a low-grade fever
(2) wheeze during inspiration
(3) be infected with parainfluenza virus
(4) show patchy areas of atelectasis on chest x-ray

384. Two weeks ago, a five-year-old boy developed diarrhea, which has persisted to the present time in spite of dietary management. His stools have been watery, pale, and frothy. He has been afebrile. Microscopic examination of his stools might show

(1) *Trichuris trichiura*
(2) *Entamoeba histolytica*
(3) *Giardia lamblia*
(4) *Toxoplasma gondii*

DIRECTIONS: The groups of questions below consist of lettered choices followed by several numbered items. For each numbered item select the **one** lettered choice with which it is **most** closely associated. Each lettered choice may be used once, more than once, or not at all.

Questions 385–386

For each of the phagocytic disorders described below, select the syndrome or disease with which it is most closely associated.

(A) Lazy leukocyte syndrome
(B) Chediak-Higashi syndrome
(C) Chronic granulomatous disease
(D) Ataxia-telangiectasia
(E) None of the above conditions

385. Abscesses, pneumonia, and osteomyelitis accompany this sex-linked or autosomal recessive condition in which leukocytes manifest normal attachment and phagocytosis but are not microbicidal for catalase-positive organisms because of defective oxidative metabolism

386. Recurrent, severe bacterial and viral infections occur in this neutropenic disorder in which leukocytes demonstrate defective chemotaxis, displayed degranulation of giant lysosomes, and normal, but delayed intracellular killing

Questions 387–390

For each of the immunologic abnormalities listed in the table below, select the syndrome or disease with which it is most closely associated.

(A) Bruton disease
(B) Di George syndrome
(C) Wiskott-Aldrich syndrome
(D) Job-Buckley syndrome
(E) Swiss-type immunodeficiency disease

	Serum IgG	Serum IgA	Serum IgM	T-Cell Function	Parathyroid Function
387.	Normal	Normal	Normal	Decreased	Decreased
388.	Low	Low	Low	Normal	Normal
389.	Low	Low	Low	Decreased	Normal
390.	Normal	High	Low	Decreased	Normal

Infectious Diseases
and Immunology
Answers

336. The answer is E. *(Behrman, ed 12. pp 399–403, 412–415.)* Rubella virus still causes congenital infections in the United States. Outbreaks occur among young adults, and there is some evidence that the number of susceptible women of childbearing age is increasing. Cytomegalovirus has become the major cause of congenital disease in this country. Fetal infection may occur in 50 percent of those pregnant women who experience a primary infection. Approximately 10 percent of these infants will develop some form of damage, such as intrauterine growth retardation, microcephaly, or deafness due to CMV. The incidence of herpes neonatorum seems to be increasing in parallel with the increase in genital herpes in the United States today. The virus becomes disseminated in two-thirds of infected infants, involving the liver, adrenals and central nervous system. The fatality rate from herpes simplex virus infection of the newborn approaches 80 percent in untreated infants. Hepatitis B virus may be transmitted to the fetus via the transplacental route or to the newborn by close contact with an infectious adult. Of those viruses mentioned, only rotavirus has not been shown to cause congenital disease.

337. The answer is B. *(Denny, J Infect Dis 123:74–92, 1971. Sanford, N Engl J Med 300:654, 656, 1979. Behrman, ed 12. pp 741–743.)* Bilateral hilar or interstitial pneumonia, especially when accompanied by a normal white blood cell count, is typical of nonbacterial disease. The picture may be confused if the patient is a coincidental carrier of pneumococci in the nasopharynx; lancet-shaped, gram-positive, α-hemolytic streptococci also may be abundantly present in pairs and resemble pneumococci. In such cases, cultures and Gram stain of tracheal aspirates are significant. Prodromal symptoms of sore throat, headache, a gradually worsening cough, and subsequent development of interstitial or hilar pneumonia are characteristic of both viral disease and *Mycoplasma pneumoniae* pneumonia, a condition highly prevalent in adolescents. Pneumonia caused by the latter agent can often be identified by specific serologic tests for *M. pneumoniae* or suggested by a significant rise in the serum cold agglutinin titer, which occurs in at least 50 percent of affected individuals.

Legionnaires' disease, caused by the gram-negative bacillus *Legionella pneumophila* is characterized by a severe bilateral interstitial pneumonia, with myalgia, headache, high fever, gastrointestinal symptoms, central nervous system dysfunction, and moderate leukocytosis and neutrophilia. Tuberculosis must be suspected if hilar adenopathy or pulmonary calicifications are present. *Mycoplasma hominis* is a genitourinary pathogen sometimes associated with postpartum fever and pelvic inflammatory disease.

338. The answer is B. *(Baraff, Pediatrics 61:224–230, 1978. Krugman, ed 7. pp 242–251. Behrman, ed 12. pp 658–661.)* Pertussis (whooping cough) should be strongly suspected in a child who, after a two-week illness resembling a common cold, develops a paroxysmal, strangling cough accompanied by profuse, thick mucus that pours from the nose and mouth. The characteristic inspiratory whoop at the end of a paroxysm, which is diagnostic for pertussis, may be absent in affected children less than six months of age. Complications include atelectasis, pneumonia, otitis media, and convulsions. Marked leukocytosis, often as high as 45,000/mm^3, with an absolute lymphocytosis is a characteristic laboratory finding. Identification of the pathogen, *Bordetella pertussis (Hemophilus pertussis)*, cannot be made by microscopic examination of secretions, except by fluorescent antibody staining techniques. Unless nasopharyngeal cultures are obtained during the first two weeks of illness or very early in the paroxysmal phase, the organism is difficult to isolate. Erythromycin is useful as prophylaxis for exposed family members and to shorten the duration of infectivity for affected infants. It does not, however, alter the course of the disease.

Because the currently available pertussis vaccine is associated with numerous side effects, the desirability of continued use of this vaccine has been discussed. However, it is clear that the public health benefits of pertussis immunization far outweigh the risks associated with pertussis immunization in young children. Recent outbreaks of pertussis (e.g., in Oklahoma) have been shown to involve children who had received inadequate immunizations.

339. The answer is E. *(Rudolph, ed 17. p 612.)* All the complications listed in the question may be associated with chickenpox except for orchitis. Inflammation of the gonads is primarily associated with infection by rubella and mumps virus. Reye's syndrome is a recently described syndrome consisting of inflammation of the central nervous system and fatty degeneration of the viscera. Reye's syndrome is also a recognized complication of influenza. Varicella encephalitis occurs less than 1 per 1000 cases of varicella. Typically, the encephalitis involves inflammation of the cerebellum. Symptoms usually begin within one week following the onset of the exanthem. Varicella pneumonia may be due to direct involvement of the lung parenchyma by the varicella virus, particularly in adults, or secondary to bacterial infection. Pneumonia as a complication of varicella has a variable course. Symptoms may be minimal or the pneumonia may be an eaarly sign of disseminated infection. Hemorrhagic varicella is a rare complication of chickenpox. This syndrome is characterized by high-grade fever and a severe chickenpox eruption associated with hemorrhage into the vesicles.

340. The answer is D. *(Feldman, Pediatrics 61:406–409, 1978. Katz, Pediatrics 55:6–8, 1975.)* Until the emergence of resistant strains of type B *Hemophilus influenzae*, intravenous ampicillin was the treatment of choice of patients who had meningitis caused by this organism. Now, however, single-agent use of intravenous chloramphenicol, which produces excellent spinal fluid levels compared with other antibiotic drugs, is recommended. To forestall the development of hemato-logic problems, ampicillin therapy can be instituted later if the causative strain is not resistant to the drug. Daily doses of ampicillin, 200–400 mg/kg, must be given to maintain adequate levels in the spinal fluid; antibiotic diffusion across the meninges diminishes as meningeal inflammation is reduced. Some authorities recommend initial therapy with both ampicillin and chloramphenicol because *H. influenzae* isolates resistant to chloramphenicol but sensitive to ampicillin have been reported. There have even been a small number of isolates resistant to both ampicillin and chloramphenicol reported in recent years. The first and second generation of cephalosporins generally do not reach therapeutic levels in the spinal fluid and cannot be used to treat meningitis. The third generation cephalosporins (cefotaxime, cefoperazone, ceftizoxime, ceftriaxone) readily penetrate the inflamed meninges and have been shown to be effective drugs in the treatment of resistant *H. influnezae* meningitis.

341. The answer is A. *(Krugman, ed 7. pp 77–89. Taylor-Robinson, N Engl J Med 302:1003–1010, 1063–1067, 1980. Behrman, ed 12. pp 653–655. Handsfield, N. Engl J Med 306:950–954, 1982.)* If vaginal or urethral discharge is present, gonococcal infection must be suspected, regardless of the affected individual's age or sexual history. Laboratory demonstration of *Neisseria gonorrhoeae* is usually but not always possible using both a Gram stain of the exudate and a culture on Thayer-Martin medium, which is more selective than chocolate agar. Gonococci can spread either hematogenously or by direct extension; infection can cause inflammation or abscess formation in the epididymis, prostate gland, fallopian tubes, peritoneal cavity, liver, and joints. Gonococcal endocarditis or meningitis, though rare, occasionally can develop. Nongonococcal urethritis accompanied by dysuria and purulent discharge, once attributed to T-stain mycoplasmas, is now thought to be caused mainly by species of *Chlamydia*. However, although this infection may be complicated by arthritis and conjunctivitis (Reiter's syndrome), meningitis does not occur. Most authorities no longer acknowledge *Mycoplasma hominis* to be a cause of symptomatic urethritis. The genital strain (type 2) of herpesvirus hominis produces a painful vesiculating balanitis or vulvitis.

Treatment of gonococcal infections has traditionally included penicillin therapy. However, since the first description in 1976 of penicillinase producing strains of *N. gonorrhoeae,* careful patient follow-up has been necessary to ensure adequate therapy. Although the incidence of penicillin resistant gonococci is low, localized outbreaks caused by resistant strains have been described in several urban areas. Resistant strains of *N. gonorrhoeae* are generally treated with either spectinomycin or newer generation cephalosporins.

342. The answer is E. *(Rudolph, ed 17. pp 592–594.)* A vesicular exanthem is not characteristic of infectious mononucleosis. To prove a diagnosis of infectious mononucleosis, a triad of findings should be present. First, physical findings may include diffuse adenopathy, tonsilar enlargement, an enlarged spleen, small hemorrhages on the soft palate, and periorbital swelling. Second, the hematologic changes should reveal a predominance of lymphocytes with at least 10 percent of these cells being atypical. Third, the characteristic antibody response should be present. Traditionally, heterophil antibodies can be detected when confirming a diagnosis of infectious mononucleosis. However, these antibodies may not be present, particularly in young children. Alternatively, specific antibodies against viral capsid antigen (VCA) on the Epstein-Barr virus may be measured. A titer of 1:152 suggests either a past infection or a recent exposure with a rising titer. Although a rash may be seen in patients with infectious mononucleosis, a vesicular exanthem is unlikely.

343. The answer is C. *(Behrman, ed 12. pp 613–615. Fleischer, Am J Dis Child 134:499–502, 1980.)* Acute osteomyelitis tends to begin abruptly with fever and marked, localized bone tenderness that usually occurs at the metaphysis. Redness and swelling frequently follow. Although usually the result of hematogenous bacterial spread, particularly of *Staphylococcus aureus,* acute osteomyelitis may follow an episode of deep cellulitis and should be suspected whenever deep cellulitis occurs. Diagnosis must often be based on clinical grounds, because bone changes may not be visible on x-ray for up to 12 days after onset of the disease. However, bone scans with technetium radioisotopes may be useful in the early diagnosis of osteomyelitis and in its differentiation from cellulitis and septic arthritis. Caution must be exercised, however, when interpreting a normal bone scan in a patient suspected of having osteomyelitis. It is clear that falsely normal bone scans do occur in patients with active bone infection. Antibiotic treatment must be initiated immediately to avoid further extension of infection into bone, where adequate drug levels are difficult to achieve. Treatment is usually continued for at least four weeks. In addition to x-rays and white blood cell count, erythrocyte sedimentation rate is useful in monitoring a patient's recovery.

344. The answer is A. *(Dodge, N Engl J Med 272: 954–960, 1003–1010, 1965. Behrman, ed 12. p 621.)* A fever accompanied by inability to flex rather than rotate the neck immediately suggests meningitis. An indolent clinical course does not rule out bacterial meningitis: *Hemophilus influenzae* may produce meningeal symptoms (fever, headache, and stiff neck or back) that are so mild that several days can elapse before medical advice is sought. The large cervical nodes characteristic of streptococcal pharyngitis may limit rotational or lateral neck movement if their tenderness is exacerbated by contraction of the sternocleidomastoid muscles. Initial symptoms of infectious mononucleosis with associated aseptic meningitis usually are pharyngitis, adenopathy (often nontender), and meningeal signs. A lumbar puncture is of prime diagnostic importance in determining the presence of bacterial meningitis, which requires immediate antibiotic therapy. A delay in treatment of even one hour may lead to such complications as cerebrovascular thrombosis, obstructive hydrocephalus, cerebritis with seizures or acute increased intracranial pressure, coma, or death.

345. The answer is E. *(Behrman, ed 12. pp 1050–1052.)* Staphylococcal pneumonia is a disease seen in patients at both ends of the age spectrum. Staphylococcal pneumonia may occur as a primary infection of the lung or as a complication of a number of viral infections such as measles, chickenpox, or influenza. Illness generally begins as an upper respiratory tract infection without specific features. The illness often progresses rapidly with the sudden onset of high fever, tachypnea, and dyspnea. Pneumatocele formation is characteristic of staphylococcal pneumonia, although it may be seen in pneumonia caused by the pneumococcus or by *Hemophilus influenzae.* Pneumothorax results when there is a rupture of a pneumatocele. Empyema results when the infection escapes the parenchyma of the lung and extends into the pleural cavity. Epiglottitis is not caused by the staphylococcus.

346. The answer is A. *(Feder, Clin Pediatr 19:457–462, 1980. Behrman, ed 12. pp 612–613, 634.)* In an infant who appears otherwise normal, the sudden onset of high fever together with a marked elevation and shift to the left of the white blood cell count suggests pneumococcal bacteremia. Viral infections such as roseola seldom cause such profound shifts in the blood leukocyte count. Streptococcosis refers to prolonged, low-grade, insidious nasopharyngitis that sometimes occurs in infants infected with group A β-hemolytic streptococci. Neither typhoid fever nor diphtheria produces markedly high white blood cell counts; both are characterized by headache, malaise, and other systemic signs. Other bacteria that should be considered in a child with this presentation include *H. influenzae* type B and the meningococcus.

347. The answer is D. *(Behrman, ed 12. p 656.)* Hemophilus influenzae, in a nonencapsulated, untypable form, can cause chronic lung disease and acute otitis media. Encapsulated strains are typed A through F, with type B being responsible for almost all of the serious infections – including meningitis, pneumonia, bacteremia, and epiglottitis – caused by this organism. The incidence of these infections increases at about the age of six months, when levels of passively transferred maternal antibody and opsonins decline, and decreases at about five years of age, presumably following repeated infections with this organism. Epidemiologic data from the Center for Disease Control for the years 1977 through 1981 indicate the relative frequency of bacterial meningitis in the United States to be as follows: *H. influenzae,* 43 percent; *N. meningitidis,* 27 percent; and *S. pneumoniae,* 11 percent.

348. The answer is A. *(Behrman, ed 12. pp 656–657, 1034–1035.)* Children who have acute epiglottitis, a life-threatening infection of the hypopharynx and epiglottis caused by *hemophilus influenzae,* typically present with high fever, extremely sore throat, and a croupy cough. Physical examination characteristically shows a red throat and a red, swollen epiglottis that may be obscured by exudate or so distorted that its identity is misinterpreted. It is important that caution be exercised while attempting to visualize the epiglottis. Abrupt glottic spasm is a well-recognized potentially fatal complication in these patients. Affected children often are unable to swallow saliva; and because the swollen epiglottis can unpredictably and suddenly cause total and fatal airway obstruction, immediate hospitalization is mandatory, even in the absence of severe respiratory distress. If a diagnosis of acute epiglottitis is uncertain, a lateral x-ray of the neck will differentiate epiglottic from subglottic swelling, the latter of which is associated with a less serious disease, croup.

349. The answer is E. *(Meissner, Pediatrics 64L348–356, 1979.)* The maximum daily dose of chloramphenicol for premature infants and for all infants during the first week of life is only 25 mg/kg. However, even this low dose can produce blood levels that exceed the therapeutic range (10 to 20 μg/ml) and suppress protein synthesis, leading to progressive lethargy, loss of sucking, a gray skin color, hypothermia, bradycardia, hypotension, and death ("gray syndrome"). Blood levels of chloramphenicol in newborn infants must be measured, regardless of the dosage, if symptoms of the gray syndrome appear. This complication has been most frequently described in infants, but the "gray toddler" syndrome – and a similar syndrome in adults – has been noted in patients with toxic levels of chloramphenicol.

350. The answer is D. *(Yow, ed 18. pp 132–133, 150, 211, 243, 305.)* The usual incubation periods of several important diseases are as follows: measles, 10 to 12 days; varicella, 10 to 21 days; rubella, 14 to 21 days; mumps, 14 to 21 days; and rabies, 9 days to several months. The durations of infectivity are as follows: measles, from the onset of the catarrhal stage through the fifth day of the rash; varicella, from one day before the eruption until the last vesicle has dried (approximately seven days); rubella, from seven days before the onset of the rash to up to eight days after its disappearance (infants with congenital rubella may excrete the virus for more than one year); mumps, from one day before until nine days after the onset of parotid swelling; and the rabies (dogs), from five days before the onset of signs through the course of the disease.

351. The answer is A. *(Behrman, ed 12. pp 747–751, 1680–1681.)* Symptoms of rubella, usually a mild disease, include a diffuse maculopapular rash that lasts for three days, marked enlargement of the posterior cervical and occipital lymph nodes, low-grade fever, mild sore throat and, occasionally, conjunctivitis, arthralgia, or arthritis. Individuals who have rubeola develop a severe cough, coryza, photophobia, conjunctivitis, and a high fever that reaches its peak at the height of the generalized macular rash, which typically lasts for five days; Koplik's spots on the buccal mucosa are diagnostic. Roseola is a viral exanthem of infants in which the high fever abruptly abates as a rash appears. Erythema infectiosum (fifth disease) begins with bright erythema on the cheeks ("slapped cheek" sign), followed by a red maculopapular rash on the trunk extremities. Erythema multiforme is a poorly understood syndrome consisting of skin lesions and mucous membrane involvement. A number of infectious agents and drugs have been associated with this syndrome.

352. The answer is C. *(Behrman, ed 12. p 745. Johnson, N Engl J Med 310:137–141, 1984.)* There are at least two forms of encephalitis associated with measles virus infection. *Postinfectious encephalitis* is the most common neurologic complication of measles and occurs about once per 1000 cases. The mortality rate may exceed 10 percent. Typically the encephalitis has its onset several days after the onset of the exanthem. Usually virus cannot be detected in brain tissue. The pathologic findings suggest an autoimmune pathogenesis. A second form of encephalitis is *subacute sclerosing panencephalitis.* This disease generally occurs in young children several years after an acute wild type measles virus infection.

353. The answer is E. *(Behrman, ed 12. p 666.)* Salmonellal gastroenteritis is usually a self-limited disease with a course rarely altered by treatment with antibiotics. Rather than eliminating the pathogen, such treatment tends to prolong the carrier state. Recommended treatment includes the administration of a diet low in roughage and fats and sufficient oral fluids to maintain blood volume and replace fecal fluid losses. Intravenous fluid hydration and maintenance, coupled with temporary discontinuation of oral intake, may be necessary in severe cases. The value of oral kaolin or pectin remains unproven. In addition to inducing the carrier state, antibiotics have *not* been found to attenuate the gastrointestinal symptoms caused by this organism. Finally, antibiotic therapy, particularly oral therapy, is likely to induce antibiotic resistance in salmonella.

354. The answer is D. *(Behrman, ed 12. pp 634–635.)* Scarlet fever results when group A β-hemolytic streptococci infecting the throat or other sites produce an erythrogenic toxin that acutely inflames the skin, kidneys, joints, or heart. The disease is easily identified by the following features: a primary site of bacterial infection, usually in the throat; a generalized, fine papular rash that has a "sandpaper" texture, is worse in the skin creases, and often involves the tongue, on which red papillae project above a thick white coat (strawberry tongue); and, following the rash, desquamation of branlike scales especially from the fingers and the tongue, causing the latter to appear red and denuded (raspberry tongue). Scarlet fever is one of the fascinating diseases that have clearly undergone a change in epidemiology and in severity in recent years. Whereas scarlet fever was formerly associated with severe sequelae, the majority of cases today are mild.

355. The answer is E. *(Rudolph, ed 17. pp 643–644.)* The incubation period for the agent of Rocky Mountain spotted fever has a range of 3 to 12 days. A brief prodromal period consisting of headache and malaise is typically followed by the abrupt onset of fever and chills. A maculopapular rash starts on the third or fourth day of illness on the flexor surfaces of the wrists and ankles before moving in a central direction. Typically, the palms and soles are involved. The rash may become hemorrhagic within one or two days. Hyponatremia may be seen in this disease, reflecting the increased permeability of the vascular system. A purulent pharyngitis is not characteristic.

356. The answer is E. *(Rudolph, ed 17. pp 625, 643, 644.)* Varicella is not generally confused with Rocky Mountain spotted fever. A morbilliform eruption may precede a petechial rash due to *Neisseria meningitidis*. In addition, septic shock is a common complication of meningococcemia. Viral infections, particularly the enteroviruses, may cause a severe illness that resembles Rocky Mountain spotted fever. In addition, several viruses have been associated with disseminated intravascular coagulation. Atypical measles is seen primarily in children who received the killed measles vaccine before 1968. After exposure to wild type measles, such a person may develop a prodrome consisting of fever, cough, headache, and myalgia. This is usually followed by the development of pneumonia and a urticarial rash beginning on the extremities. Toxic shock syndrome (TSS) is a disease characterized by sudden onset of fever, diarrhea, shock, mucous membrane inflammation, and a diffuse macular rash resulting in desquamation of the hands and feet. Fluid loss with shock is a common complication. TSS occurs most commonly in menstruating women and appears to be associated with the presence of a toxin-producing strain of *S. aureus* in the vagina.

357. The answer is C. *(Behrman, ed 12. p 584.)* The combination of erythema multiforme and vesicular, ulcerated lesions of the mucous membranes of the eyes, mouth, anus, and urethra defines the Stevens-Johnson syndrome (erythema multiforme exudativum). Fever is common and pulmonary involvement occasionally is noted; the mortality rate can approach 10 percent. Common complications include corneal ulceration, dehydration due to severe stomatitis and subsequently poor fluid intake, and urinary retention caused by dysuria. Among the known causes of the Stevens-Johnson syndrome are allergy to various drugs (including barbiturates, sulfonamides, and penicillin) and infection with *Mycoplasma pneumoniae*.

358. The answer is E. *(Meissner, Pediatrics 64:348–356, 1976.)* Aplastic anemia induced by chloramphenicol is relatively uncommon (1 case in every 60,000 to 100,000 individuals receiving the drug). It has been estimated that the incidence of chloramphenicol-induced aplastic anemia occurs at about the same incidence as death due to penicillin anaphylaxis. Not usually dose-related, it is an idiosyncratic reaction that can occur either during therapy or up to many months after; it usually has a fatal outcome. In contrast, chloramphenicol-induced bone marrow suppression is extremely common, is dose-related, occurs during therapy, and responds satisfactorily to a reduction in dose or cessastion of treatment.

359.   The answer is A. *(Fekety, Rev Inf Dis 5:246-257, 1983.) Bacillus cereus* is an important cause of diarrhea after ingestion of improperly cooked rice in Oriental restaurants. Enterotoxigenic *E. coli* is the major cause of diarrhea in U.S. travelers to tropical areas. *Yersinia enterocolitica* is being recognized with greater frequency as an important cause of diarrhea in this country due to improvement in isolation techniques. *Campylobacter jejuni* in many studies is as important a cause of diarrhea as *Salmonella.*

360.   The answer is B. *(Dillon, Am J Dis Child 115:530–541, 1968. Behrman, ed 12. pp 752, 758–759, 1711–1712. Peter, N Engl J Med 297:311–317, 1977.)* Streptococcal impetigo is a superficial pyoderma in which thin-walled vesicles rupture very rapidly, creating oozing or crusted honey-colored sores; these sores may be the first lesions noted by an affected individual. The vesicles of staphylococcal impetigo are more durable and may not rupture as the lesions spread. Impetigo is usually painless; painful, crusted, spreading lesions on the face are ordinarily caused by herpesvirus hominis, type 1, which also can cause a distinctive, painful, red swelling of a fingertip with clusters of thick wall vesicles. Herpes zoster infection features painful vesicles in a linear arrangement along dermatomes. Staphylococcal impetigo most frequently develops in neonates in the periumbilical area, whereas impetigo contagiosa is primarily an endemic disease of pre-school-age children.

361.   The answer is B (1, 3). *(Thompson, Pediatrics 66:936–942, 1980.)* Infant botulism is a neuromuscular disease caused by the toxin of *Clostridium botulinum.* The disease is distinct from classic botulism in that spores are ingested and the toxin is synthesized by the organism while it resides in the infant's intestine. The toxin is then absorbed and produces weakness and paralysis because of impaired release of acetylcholine at the neuromuscular synapse. Recent evidence suggests a broad clinical spectrum of infant botulism. Some infants may never require hospitalization and demonstrate only minimal feeding difficulties. More severely affected infants may have a presentation that suggests the sudden infant death syndrome. Infants who survive show a complete resolution of symptoms.

362.   The answer is B (1, 3). *(Krugman, ed 7. pp 162–167, 462. Behrman, ed 12. pp 625–626.)* The aseptic meningitis syndrome refers to a variety of disorders characterized by meningitis associated with a conspicuous number of lymphocytes but no organisms visible on Gram stain. Causes include infections with viruses, rickettsiae, spirochetes, fungi, protozoa, and mycobacteria. Among noninfectious causes are tumors, leukemia, poisons such as lead, and meningeal irritation from intrathecally injected material, contiguous lesions, or allergy. In contrast to the typically low cerebrospinal fluid (CSF) glucose levels (less than half the blood glucose level) in bacterial meningitis, the CSF glucose level in aseptic meningitis ordinarily is normal. Important exceptions include infections with *Mycobacterium tuberculosis* and fungi, which usually produce low CSF glucose levels; virus infections very rarely depress the CSF glucose level. Once suspected, tubercle bacilli can be visualized by an acid-fast stain, and the yeast *Cryptococcus neoformans* (torula) by an india-ink preparation. The presence of minute amounts of alcohol in the CSF results from the fermentation of glucose and indicates the presence of the fungi.

363. The answer is A (1, 2, 3). *(Kohl, Pediatr Clin North Am 26:433–443, 1979. Prince, Pediatr Clin North Am 26:261–268, 1979. Steinhoff, J Pediatr 96:611–622, 1980. Torphy, Pediatrics 64:898–903, 1979.)* *Yersinia enterocolitica* is a gram-negative, invasive member of the Enterobacteriaceae family. As the etiologic agent of one form of prolonged diarrhea, with vomiting, fever, and abdominal pain that may resemble acute appendicitis, it is rarely identified by routine bacteriologic cultures. Because it can be isolated easily with special bacteriologic techniques, some authorities predict that *Y. enterocolitica* will prove to be an important cause of common-source outbreaks of gastroenteritis. Human rotavirus infection is characterized by winter outbreaks of sudden vomiting, fever, and diarrhea, often accompanied by upper respiratory tract symptoms. It may affect both adults and children within families and appears to be the single most important etiologic agent in childhood gastroenteritis. *Campylobacter fetus* (formerly *Vibrio fetus*) is emerging as an important cause of both common-source and sporadic diarrhea. The enteritis commonly is associated with severe abdominal cramps and diarrheal stools, which may contain blood or mucus. In addition to enteritis, at least two other patterns of human disease occur with infection with this pathogen: bacteremia and focal infections in older, debilitated men, and perinatal infections of mothers or infants. Special bacteriologic techniques are required to isolate this organism. During either oral or parenteral therapy with antibiotics, particularly ampicillin, penicillin, and clindamycin, the normal bowel flora are markedly reduced in number, allowing proliferation of *Clostridium difficile*. This bacteria elaborates a toxin which then produces profuse watery diarrhea, fever, vomiting, and abdominal distension, with typical pseudomembranous plaques visible by proctoscopy. This syndrome, known as antibiotic-associated pseudomembranous colitis, usually remits when the antibiotic is stopped but may in some cases progress to toxic megacolon, peritonitis, and shock. In such cases, intravenous fluid replacement and eradication of the clostridia with vancomycin may be life-threatening.

364. The answer is B (1, 3). *(Krugman, ed 7. pp 4–8, 417–425.)* Microcephaly accompanied by intracranial calcification, particularly in the ventricular ependyma, is highly characteristic of congenital toxoplasmosis or infection with cytomegalovirus. Definitive diagnosis of either disease may be made by demonstration of a rising antibody titer to either pathogen; in addition, cytomegalovirus can be cultured from the urine of affected individuals. It is important to note that maternal immunoglobulin G antibodies may passively cross the placenta and initially produce positive serologic titers in the newborn for *Toxoplasma, Treponema,* cytomegalovirus, or rubella. Therefore, to document that an antibody is of fetal origin, a stable or rising antibody titer must be demonstrated or the nondiffusable immunoglobulin M antibody fraction must be tested.

365. The answer is A (1,2,3). *(Sullivan, Adv Pediatr 31:365–399, 1984.)* The Epstein-Barr virus has one of the longest incubation periods of any conventional virus. Once an individual has been infected by the Epstein-Barr virus, the virus is carried in B lymphocytes for the life of the host. Periodically, the virus is excreted from B lymphocytes into the saliva of the infected host. At any one point, 15 percent of seropositive individuals will excrete the virus in their saliva. When a seronegative individual comes in contact with EBV-containing saliva, a primary infection may occur. Once a person has had a primary EBV infection, a fresh infection by an exogenous virus does not occur. However, there may be reactivation of the endogenous Epstein-Barr virus infection under certain circumstances when the latent virus is permitted to reactivate.

366. The answer is B (1, 3). *(Lumicao, Pediatr Clin North Am 26:269–282, 1979. Tipple, Pediatrics 63:192–197, 1979.)* Chlamydial species include *Chlamydia psittaci* and *Chlamydia trachomatis,* both of which are pathogenic for humans. *C. psittaci* causes ornithosis, an infection ordinarily contracted from birds, principally parrots, parakeets, turkeys, and ducks. Ornithosis is characterized by interstitial pneumonia, fever, headache, and myalgias. Much more prevalent are infections with various serotypes of *C. trachomatis,* which cause trachoma, chlamydial conjunctivitis of the newborn, chlamydial pneumonia of infancy, nongonococcal and postgonococcal urethritis, and lymphogranuloma venereum. Chlamydial conjunctivitis of the newborn (inclusion blenorrhea) can be differentiated from other causes of neonatal conjunctivitis by the time of onset and by culture and stain techniques. In contrast to the chemical conjunctivitis produced by silver nitrate eye drops, which occurs within the first two days of life, and to bacterial conjunctivitis, which often develops within the first week of life and which can be identified with routine bacteriologic cultures and Gram stain, inclusion blenorrhea typically appears at approximately 10 to 14 days of life. The characteristic inclusion bodies may be seen within the cytoplasm of epithelial cells obtained by conjunctival swabbing and Giemsa staining. Chlamydial pneumonia of infancy usually occurs between one and three months of age and develops gradually. Characterized clinically by a frequent and persistent cough, tachypnea, inspiratory rales, normal temperature, and a chest x-ray pattern of interstitial infliltrates and hyperinflation, the illness tends to continue for several weeks. Lymphogranduloma venereum (LGV) is a sexually transmitted disease caused by three relatively invasive serotypes of *C. trachomatis*. Following the production of a primary lesion on the genitals or urethra, a second stage occurs, with tender enlargement of the regional lymph nodes, often accompanied by a fever. A third stage, with tissue destruction leading to rectal strictures, may occur.

367. The answer is E (all). *(Krugman, ed 7. pp 7–8, 322–326, 395–399, 421–423. Behrman, ed 12. pp 399–401, 411–413, 848.)* Sepsis of the newborn may first manifest as jaundice and thrombocytopenic purpura. Among the important causes of neonatal sepsis are prenatal infections, including congenital syphilis, toxoplasmosis, cytomegalic inclusion disease, and rubella. Useful diagnostic studies, in addition to cultures for bacteria, include specific serologic tests for pathogens, viral cultures for cytomegalovirus, lumbar puncture, x-rays of the chest and long bones, and measurement of the cord-blood immunoglobulin M level, which often is increased in prenatal infections. Longitudinal striations in the metaphyses are characteristic of congenital rubella, while osteochondritis or periostitis usually indicates congenital syphilis. Congenital syphilis, cytomegalovirus disease, and rubella may be highly contagious. Urine may contain rubella virus for more than six months and is therefore a special hazard to nonimmune pregnant women.

368. The answer is C (2, 4). *(Hoekelman, pp 777–781. Seto, Pediatr Clin North Am 26:305–314, 1979.)* Hepatitis A (infectious hepatitis) is characterized by a relatively short incubation period (15 to 50 days) following transmission of the virus, primarily by the fecal-oral route. Its onset is abrupt, with sudden fever, nausea, vomiting, anorexia, and liver tenderness, soon followed by jaundice. Elevated serum levels of bilirubin and aspartate aminotransferase (glutamic-oxaloacetic transaminase, SGOT) are transient, usually not persisting more than three weeks. Viremia is brief and the period of maximum infectivity of stools usually occurs during the two-week period prior to the onset of jaundice. Hepatitis B (serum hepatitis), usually transmitted parenterally via blood or blood products, may also be transmitted nonparenterally via body fluids such as saliva or semen. Following a long incubation period (40 to 180 days), there is gradual onset of low fever, anorexia, and jaundice, often preceded or accompanied by extrahepatic manifestations such as macular rashes, arthralgias, or urticaria, which may mimic serum sickness. Serum levels of SGOT and bilirubin may be elevated for months, the latter sometimes rising to levels greater than 20 mg/100 ml when associated with the fulminant hepatitis more often seen with hepatitis B infection. Viremia usually persists throughout the clinical course of hepatitis B infections and may progress to a chronic carrier state in 10 percent of individuals, most of whom are asymptomatic. These may be identified by the persistence of the viral surface antigen HB_s Ag in their blood. A third type of hepatitis is referred to as non-A, non-B hepatitis, reflecting the likelihood that more than one additional virus may cause this syndrome. Non-A, non-B hepatitis is important because it accounts for 80 to 90 percent of posttransfusion hepatitis in the United States. In addition, it is associated with a high rate of chronicity (25 to 50 percent).

369. The answer is D (4). *(Blacklow, N Engl J Med 304:397–406, 1981.)* Adults are frequently infected with rotavirus. Asymptomatic rotavirus infections can occur in adult contacts. Parents of infants infected with rotavirus may have diarrhea and abdominal cramps. In addition, rotavirus is a recognized cause of travelers' diarrhea in both children and adults. Rotavirus is the most common cause of diarrhea among hospitalized children. The virus is often detected in feces for up to eight days after the onset of disease. It is a major cause of nosocomical diarrhea among hospitalized pediatric patients. In contrast to many other causes of acute gastroenteritis, rotavirus-induced disease is frequently associated with vomiting. Infected children are most commonly between 6 and 24 months of age.

370. The answer is E (all). *(Hopkins, JAMA 210:694–700, 1969. Krugman, ed 7. pp 556–559. Behrman, ed 12. pp 191, 661, 746, 762–763.)* Encephalitis is a rare but serious complication of immunization with smallpox, pertussis, and measles vaccines. It occurs most commonly following smallpox vaccination (1 case per 100,000 in the United States, up to 1 case per 4000 in Europe, with a mortality rate of 50 percent). The incidence of encephalitis following live measles vaccination may approach 3 cases for every 1 million children vaccinated. Pertussis antigen must not be given to a child who has a history of convulsions following previous exposure to pertussis vaccine. Simple febrile convulsions following administration of these three vaccines are not rare in susceptible children less than three years of age. Development of poliomyelitis following trivalent oral polio vaccination occurs less often than 1 child per 10 million apparently normal children. A greater risk, however, occurs for adults, both those in contact with vaccinated children and those being vaccinated themselves; it is advised, therefore, that adults should not be vaccinated routinely. Live-virus vaccines should not be used in immunosuppressed individuals.

371. The answer is B (1, 3). *(Sullivan, Adv Pediatr 31:365–399, 1984.)* One disadvantage of the heterophil test is that some pediatric patients do not manifest heterophil antibodies in response to an Epstein-Barr virus infection. Even in adults, heterophil antibodies may not be detectable for two to three weeks after the onset of illness. A differential heterophil assay will differentiate between serum sickness and infectious mononucleosis. Because heterophil antibodies may persist for up to 18 months in some patients, it may be difficult to decide if the positive heterophils reflect an acute infection or an infection some time in the past. Antibodies directed against the viral capsid antigen on the Epstein-Barr virus will persist for the life of the host. IgM antibodies against this antigen are invariably present early in infection

372. The answer is C (2, 4). *(Behrman, ed 12. pp 403–405.)* The prodromal features of bacterial meningitis during the first six months of life may be very subtle; symptoms may include lethargy and anorexia. High fever may not occur, but when present during this period, it is an extremely important sign of sepsis; urine and blood cultures and a lumbar puncture should be performed. The classic indications of meningitis — fever, stiff neck, bulging fontanelle, high-pitched cry, vomiting, and convulsions — may be absent in small infants who have the disease. In the differential diagnosis of fever in children less than six months of age, streptococcal pharyngitis and roseola infantum are extremely unusual; urinary tract infections, however, must be considered carefully and are often associated with congenital anomalies involving the urinary tract.

373. The answer is E (all). *(Behrman, ed 12. pp 743–746.)* Measles is a generalized viral infection that can affect many organ systems. The disease characteristically is heralded by a severe respiratory infection that produces a harsh cough, profuse clear nasal discharge, red conjunctivae, photophobia, and high fever. A widespread, blotchy, red rash appears on the fourth or fifth day, and the symptoms worsen as the rash spreads. The rash and other symptoms abate in approximately five days. Koplik's spots on the buccal mucosa are pathognomonic. Complications of measles that are often encountered include encephalitis, primary viral or secondary bacterial pneumonia, viral myocarditis, group A β-hemolytic streptococci, pharyngitis or otitis media, and thrombocytopenic purpura with hemorrhages into the skin ("black measles"). It should be noted that the incidence of measles in the United States is falling dramatically as a result of the widespread use of the measles vaccine. During 1982, slightly fewer than 1700 cases of measles were reported to the Center for Disease Control.

374. The answer is A (1, 2, 3). *(Behrman, ed 12. pp 1719–1721.)* Infection caused by *Candida albicans* ranges from a superficial mucocutaneous infection such as thrush to disseminated disease such as that occuring in newborns or patients receiving immunotherapy. Newborn infants may acquire the yeast during passage through a colonized birth canal. Final proof of invasive disease requires the demonstration of pseudohyphal forms in infected tissues. Chronic mucocutaneous candidiasis is a specific syndrome associated with immunologic defects and endocrinopathies. Amphotricin B remains the drug of choice when intravenous therapy is necessary for invasive disease.

375. The answer is E (all). *(Behrman, ed 12. pp 1710–1711. Yow, ed 18, pp 285–299.)* Allergic response to tubercle bacilli is the basis for the intracutaneous Mantoux test for tuberculosis; the test becomes positive within two to ten weeks after infection. Cross-reactions to atypical mycobacteria sometimes occur and can be differentiated from positive reactions for tuberculosis by the relatively larger intradermal reaction to the specific atypical antigen. The Mantoux test may become negative either during advanced stages of tuberculosis or briefly after immunization with live-virus vaccines (such as measles, rubella, and smallpox), administration of corticosteroids or immunosuppressive durgs, or development of a febrile illness or dehydration. Except in regions where atypical mycobacterial disease is endemic, a positive skin test in a child warrants antimicrobial therapy for at least one year. Explanations for a false negative skin test in a patient with tuberculosis include overwhelming tuberculous infection, recent infection by or vaccination against measles virus (resulting in anergy), or methodologic problems associated with placing the skin test.

376. The answer is A (1, 2, 3). *Hoekelman, pp 1012, 1014.)* In a black child with the typical features of acute osteomyelitis depicted in the x-ray that accompanies the question (periosteal new bone formation and cortical destruction involving the fourth metatarsal bone), underlying sickle cell disease should be strongly suspected. Because of the increased frequency of osteomyelitis due to *Salmonella* and other encapsulated organisms in patients with sickle cell disease, initial therapy should include an antibiotic with known effectiveness against that organism. Many patients with sickle cell disease eventually develop functional hyposplenism and thus have a high incidence of pneumococcal bacteremia. Accordingly, prophylactic administration of polyvalent pneumococcal vaccine is recommended.

377. The answer is E (all). *(Meissner, Am J Dis Child 136:465–467, 1982.)* Lyme disease is characterized by a unique skin lesion, recurrent attacks of arthritis, and occasional involvement of the heart and central nervous system. Illness usually appears in late summer or early fall, one to two weeks after a bite by an infecting tick. Erythema chronicum migrans begins as a red macule usually on the trunk at the site of tick attachment. Nonspecific systemic signs include headache, fever, and malaise. Joint involvement generally occurs three to four weeks after onset of the rash. Cardiac disease consists primarily of rhythm disturbances. CNS involvement is evidenced by headache and stiff neck. Treatment with penicillin does result in a faster resolution of symptoms.

378. The answer is E (all). *(Behrman, ed 12. pp 793–795.)* Poliomyelitis infection, though familiarly paralytic, also can be asymptomatic, producing only a brief viremia after the virus has multiplied in the intestinal tract. In both the nonparalytic and paralytic varieties, fever, sore throat, muscle pains, and aseptic meningitis with nuchal rigidity are prominent features. Complications include gastric ulcers, hypertension, bladder paralysis, and respiratory paralysis. Polio will continue to occur sporadically as long as lax immunization practices persist.

379. The answer is E (all). *(Behrman, ed 12. pp 651–652.)* Meningococcemia may be complicated by a variety of septic disorders, including meningitis, purulent pericarditis, endocarditis, pneumonia, otitis media, and arthritis. (Arthritis associated with meningococcemia may be mediated by an immune mechanism rather than bacterial invasion of the joint.) The potent endotoxin of the causative organism, *Neisseria meningitidis,* can induce shock, disseminated intravascular coagulation with associated hemorrhaging, and acute adrenal failure caused by localized intraadrenal bleeding; these reactions can be collectively referred to as the Waterhouse-Friderichsen syndrome. Vaccines against *N. meningitidis* group A and C are now available, but they fail to protect young infants, who comprise a majority of the civilian population at risk. Prophylaxis with rifampin or minocycline for persons in close contact with affected individuals is recommended by many authorities.

380. The answer is A (1, 2, 3). *(Behrman, ed 12. pp 618–626.)* In individuals who have meningitis, a glucose level in the cerebrospinal fluid that is less than 50 percent of the blood glucose level suggests a bacterial, fungal, mycobacterial, or occasionally viral infection. Early in the course of bacterial meningitis, the white blood cell count in cerebrospinal fluid may be difficult to interpret; within hours however, the characteristically high percentage (90 percent) of polymorphonuclear leukocytes appears. In mild, equivocal cases (leukocyte count less than 1000/mm³), antibiotic treatment might well be delayed pending a second lumbar puncture four to six hours after the initial tap. Awareness of an increased incidence of aseptic meningitis in the community may offer an additional reason for a delay in antibiotic therapy until a second lumbar puncture is performed several hours later. If this course is chosen, the patient must be carefully followed for any deterioration in condition. Nonbacterial meningitis that has developed in association with an illness causing submandibular or cervical swelling suggests mumps or infectious mononucleosis; abnormal serum amylase concentration or heterophil agglutinaton test results, respectively, are diagnostic.

381. The answer is A (1, 2, 3). *(Behrman, ed 12. pp 854–861.)* Ascaris lumbricoides larvae travel through the intestinal wall and end up, by way of the liver, in the lungs, where they commonly produce pneumonia and peripheral eosinophilia (Loffler's syndrome); worms mature in the small intestine, where they sometimes cause obstruction. The larvae of *Toxocara canis* migrate from the intestine to all parts of the body, where granulomatous reactions may occur (visceral larva migrans). Hookworms *(Necator americanus)* can cause intestinal blood loss from mucosal laceration; cutaneous larva migrans occurs when hookworm larvae fail to enter cutaneous blood vessels after penetrating the skin. Pinworms *(Enterobius vermicularis)* develop only in the colon, producing no internal disease other than a rare case of appendicitis. However, gravid worms crawl out of the anus at night, disturbing sleep and causing severe pruritus. Vaginitis and salpingitis may occur if the worms then enter the vagina.

382. The answer is E (all). *(Krugman, ed 7. pp 366–367, 370, 372–373. Behrman ed 12. pp 410–411.)* Colonization of a newborn infant with *Staphylococcus aureus* commonly occurs either through the skin or by way of the umbilicus, the latter leading to a purulent drainage that progresses to local redness and swelling. Although the resulting dermatitis is usually pustular, it occasionally may appear as pemphigus neonatorum, which is characterized by bulla formation, or as the "scalded skin syndrome," which features generalized erythema, tenderness, and exfoliation, especially after stroking (Nikolsky's sign). Staphylococcal neonatal mastitis is associated with a progressive enlargement of one or both breasts beyond the normal hypertrophy often noted at birth. In a newborn infant, osteomyelitis, which usually is staphylococcal causes pseudoparalysis or point tenderness over a long bone; staphylococcal pneumonia and meningitis also can develop. Fever and other clinical signs of systemic sepsis may not be present in infants who have staphylococcal infections.

383. The answer is B (1, 3). *(Behrman, ed 12. pp 1034–1037.)* Croup, an infection of early childhood, involves the larynx and trachea; it usually is caused by parainfluenza or respiratory syncytial viruses. Symptoms include a low-grade fever, barking cough, and hoarse inspiratory stridor without wheezing. The pharynx may be normal or slightly red, and the lungs usually are clear. In children in severe respiratory distress, prolonged dyspnea can progress to physical exhaustion and fatal respiratory failure. Because agitation may be a sign of hypoxia, sedation should not be ordered.

384. The answer is A (1, 2, 3). *(Behrman, ed 12. pp 837, 847–850.)* Persistent, nonsuppurative diarrhea can be caused by amebas, whipworms (trichuriasis), or *Giardia lamblia.* Amebas produce an ulcerating colitis that may be very mild or extremely destructive. Amebic liver abscess should be suspected when fever, chills, leukocytosis, and right upper quadrant pain or tenderness follow diarrhea. Whipworm infection can lead to chronic irritation of the bowel wall and thus to diarrhea and rectal prolapse. Diarrhea associated with giardiasis probably occurs because of malabsorption resulting from extensive coating of intestinal mucosa by the parasite. Infestation often results from contaminated municipal or well water and is accompanied by intermittent abdominal cramps and flatulence, as well as by prolonged diarrhea. Acquired *Toxoplasma gondii* can infest any body tissue, resulting in fever, myalgia, lymphadenopathy, maculopapular rash, hepatomegaly, pneumonia, encephalitis, chorioretinitis, and mycarditis. This intracellular parasite does not ordinarily cause diarrhea and is not found in stools. Congenital toxoplasmosis may occur if a mother first acquires the parasite during pregnancy. Her infected newborn infant may demonstrate jaundice, hepatosplenomegaly, hydrocephalus or microcephaly, intracranial calcification, or chorioretinitis.

385–386. The answers are: 385-C, 386-B. *(Hoekleman, pp 1068–1069. Behrman, ed 12. pp 519–523.)* Disorders of leukocytes include (1) defective locomotion out of the bone marrow, (2) depressed chemotaxis involving cellular defects, chemotactic inhibitors, or deficiencies of chemotactic factors, and (3) inability to ingest or kill microorganisms. Sometimes several disorders are present concurrently. *Defective locomotion* results in the neutropenia characteristic of the lazy leukocyte syndrome, in which abnormal chemotaxis, otitis media, and stomatitis are also part of the clinical picture. *Depressed cellular chemotaxis* is associated with the Job-Buckley syndrome (hyperimmunoglobulin E, eczema, and recurrent staphylococcal infections), Down's syndrome, and the Chediak-Higashi syndrome (see below), among others. Inhibition of chemotaxis is seen in association with excesses of certain plasma proteins, including IgA. These excesses sometimes occur with rheumatoid arthiritis, the Wiskott-Aldrich syndrome, and Hodgkin's disease. Deficiency of chemotactic factors, most of which are components of the complement system, may in association with deficient levels of complement produce recurrent, severe infections caused by encapsulated bacteria. Among the diseases associated with the *inability of leukocytes to kill ingested microorganisms* is chronic granulomatous disease, sex linked in 80 percent of cases. In individuals so affected, severe recurrent pneumonia and abscesses of lymph nodes and of the liver are caused by a variety of catalase-positive bacteria. These can survive ingestion by the defective leukocytes which lack normal oxidative metabolism and cannot produce microbicidal superoxide and hydrogen peroxide. These leukocytes can be identified in the laboratory by their failure to reduce nitroblue tetrazolium (NBT tests). Chediak-Higashi syndrome, caused by another leukocyte defect, is characterized by abnormally large intracytoplasmic lysosomes, visible as giant granules (Dohl bodies), which degranulate in a delayed manner after phagocytosis of pathogens. Thus, oxidative metabolism and consequent microbial killing are delayed. Neutropenia, depressed chemotaxis, and recurrent pyogenic infections are accompanying abnormalities.

387–390. The answers are: 387-B, 388-A, 389-E, 390-C. *(Hoekleman, pp 1065–1068. Behrman, ed 12. pp 504–511, 522.)* Many primary immunologic deficiencies may be classified as defects of T-lymphocyte function (containment of fungi, protozoa, acid-fast bacteria, and certain viruses) and B-lymphocyte function (synthesis and secretion of immunoglobulins). Among the T-cell diseases is the Di George syndrome in which defective embryologic development of the third and fourth pharyngeal pouches results in hypoplasia of both thymus and parathyroid glands. Primary B-cell diseases include panhypogammaglobulinemia *(Bruton disease)*, an X-linked deficiency of all three major classes of immunoglobulins, as well as other selective deficiencies of the immunoglobulins or their subgroups. Combined T- and B-cell diseases include the X-linked *Wiskott-Aldrich syndrome* of mild T-cell dysfuncton, diminished serum IgM, marked elevation of IgA and IgE, eczema, recurrent middle ear infections, and thrombocytopenia. Patients with the catastrophic combined T- and B-cell disease known as combined immuno-deficiency disease *(Swiss-type lymphopenic agammaglobulinemia)* lack function-ing T and B cells. Consequently, there are both marked lymphopenia and agammaglobulinemia, as well as hypoplasia of the thymus. Chronic diarrhea, rashes, recurrent serious bacterial, fungal, or viral infections, wasting, and early death are characteristic. Other T- and B-cell deficiencies include ataxia-telangiectasia and chronic mucocutaneous candidiasis. *Job-Buckley syndrome* is a disorder of phagocyte cell chemotaxis associated with hypergammaglobulin E, eczema, and recurrent severe staphylococcal infections.

Hematologic and Neoplastic Diseases

Shiao Y. Woo

DIRECTIONS: Each question below contains five suggested answers. Choose the **one best** response to each question.

391. Thrombocytopenia in the newborn can be associated with all of the following EXCEPT

(A) congenital cytomegalovirus infection
(B) perinatal aspiration syndrome
(C) maternal idiopathic thrombocytopenic purpura (ITP)
(D) maternal ingestion of aspirin
(E) absence of radii in the infant

392. The most common cause of death in children who have homozygous β-thalassemia is

(A) hepatic insufficiency
(B) diabetes mellitus
(C) cardiac arrhythmias and congestive heart failure
(D) overwhelming bacterial sepsis
(E) hypoadrenalism

393. A 15-month-old boy presents with recurrent furuncles for a duration of three months. He has not had any serious infection that requires hospitalization. Physical examination reveals a few palpable cervical and inguinal lymph nodes and two furuncles at the perirectal region. His white count is 5100/mm^3 with a differential of 6 percent polymorphonuclear neutrophils, 3 percent monocytes, and 1 percent eosinophils and 90 percent lymphocytes. The LEAST likely diagnosis is

(A) cyclic neutropenia
(B) benign childhood neutropenia
(C) Kostman's syndrome
(D) dilantin therapy
(E) acute leukemia

394. The spleen indisputably shortens red blood cell survival in which of the following conditions?

(A) Pyruvate kinase deficiency
(B) Hexokinase deficiency
(C) Glucose-6-phosphate dehydrogenase deficiency
(D) Hereditary spherocytosis
(E) Acquired idiopathic hemolytic anemia

395. A six-month-old infant presents with failure to thrive, psychomotor deterioration, and hepatosplenomegaly. Wright-Giemsa staining of a bone marrow aspirate shows large numbers of cells, as illustrated below. These findings are associated most closely with

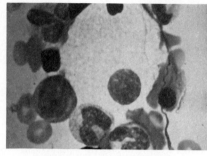

- (A) histiocytosis X
- (B) Gaucher's disease
- (C) Niemann-Pick disease
- (D) Hurler's syndrome
- (E) myelogenous leukemia

396. A ten-year-old boy is admitted to the hospital because of bleeding. Pertinent laboratory findings include a platelet count of 50,000/mm³, prothrombin time (PT) of 15 s (control 11.5 s), activated partial thromboplastin time (aPTT) of 51 s (control 36 s), thrombin time (TT) 13.7 s (control 10.5 s), and factor VIII level 14% (normal 38–178%). The most likely cause of his bleeding is

- (A) idiopathic thrombocytopenic purpura (ITP)
- (B) hemophilia A
- (C) disseminated intravascular coagulation (DIC)
- (D) liver disease
- (E) vitamin K deficiency

397. In the long-term treatment of iron overload in children with homozygous thalassemia, the most effective iron chelation is accomplished when deferoxamine (Desferol) is given by

- (A) mouth
- (B) intramuscular injection
- (C) intravenous infusion
- (D) subcutaneous infusion
- (E) subcutaneous infusion with vitamin C supplementation

398. At 12 hours of age, a polycythemic infant looks anxious, sweaty, and jittery. The most important part of the definitive treatment of this child's hematologic disorder should be

- (A) phlebotomy
- (B) phlebotomy followed by replacement with normal saline
- (C) infusion of normal saline
- (D) a partial plasma exchange transfusion
- (E) institution of intravenous glucose therapy

399. A six-year-old girl is hospitalized because of pallor and fatigue of a few weeks duration. When she was 18 months of age, she had iron deficiency anemia that responded to oral iron and blood transfusion therapy; at that time a stool guaiac of 3 was attributed to excessive milk intake. When she was four years of age, her anemia recurred; treatment with intramuscular iron was effective. Except for her pallor, physical examination is unremarkable. Laboratory results are hemoglobin, 5 g/100 ml; reticulocytes, 3%; and microcytic, hypochronic erythrocytes in the peripheral blood smear. Neither the child nor her parents have been aware of her having gastrointestinal symptoms or blood in the stools.

The cause of this child's anemia would best be established by

(A) screening for sickle cell hemoglobin
(B) testing for serum iron and total iron-binding capacity
(C) a hemolytic workup
(D) a barium study of the gastrointestinal tract
(E) a red blood cell survival test (^{51}chromium labeling)

400. All of the following statements are associated with children and adolescents with sickle cell anemia EXCEPT that

(A) height and weight are reduced as compared with national health statistic norms
(B) bone age is delayed
(C) there is delayed sexual maturation
(D) the plasma concentrations of pituitary gonadotropin do not rise during puberty
(E) the incidence of cholelithiasis increases during adolescence

401. A 10-year old boy who has moderately severe hemophilia A and is on a home treatment program has just suffered a mild spontaneous hemorrhage into his right knee joint. Knowing that infusion of 1 unit of factor VIII per kg body weight raises the plasma factor VIII level by 2 percent with a subsequent half-life of 12 hours, what level should be attained for adequate initial control?

(A) 5 to 10 percent of normal
(B) 10 to 20 percent of normal
(C) 20 to 30 percent of normal
(D) 30 to 40 percent of normal
(E) 40 to 50 precent of normal

402. The following statements concerning side effects of antineoplastic agents are true EXCEPT that

(A) vincristine can cause peripheral neuropathy
(B) prednisone can cause alopecia
(C) methotrexate can cause mucositis
(D) 6-mercaptopurine can cause hepatic dysfunction
(E) adriamycin (doxorubicin) can cause cardiomyopathy

403. The value of free erythrocyte prophyrin:hemoglobin ratio (FEP:Hg) is usually abnormal in all of the following conditions EXCEPT

(A) early, mild iron deficiency anemia
(B) severe iron deficiency anemia
(C) α- or β-thalassemia trait
(D) lead poisoning
(E) erythropoietic protoporphyria

404. Granulocyte transfusions are most likely to be effective in which of the following patients with acute leukemia?

(A) A neutropenic patient in remission with documented septicemia
(B) A neutropenic patient in remission with *Pneumocystis carinii* infection
(C) A neutropenic patient in relapse with undocumented infection
(D) A patient with refractory acute leukemia with infection and pancytopenia
(E) A patient in remission following bone marrow transplantation

405. Premature infants three to six months of age and older are more prone to develop significant anemia than are comparably aged full-term infants. This late anemia of prematurity is most likely to be the consequence of

(A) a lack of erythropoietin synthesis
(B) a decreased oxygen requirement and an increased oxygen unloading capacity
(C) decreased red blood cell survival
(D) rapid growth and diminished iron reserves
(E) poor utilization of available iron in food

406. During the last 30 years, the two-year disease-free survival rate of children who have Wilms' tumor has improved from 30 to 90 percent. Which of the following therapeutic factors have contributed most to this increased survival rate?

(A) Improved surgical techniques
(B) A megavoltage apparatus during radiation therapy
(C) Actinomycin D
(D) Vincristine
(E) Actinomycin D and vincristine in combination

407. Neuroblastoma can be associated with all of the following statements EXCEPT that

(A) approximately 50 percent of neuroblastomas occur during the first two years of life
(B) heterochromia iridis and Horner's syndrome may be manifestations of cervical neuroblastoma
(C) metastases are uncommon at the time of diagnosis
(D) serial measurements of urinary catecholamines are useful in predicting the progression of neuroblastoma
(E) spontaneous regression is known to occur in neuroblastoma

408. All of the following statements regarding Hodgkin's disease are true EXCEPT that

(A) Hodgkin's disease is very rare below the age of five years, but there is a peak of incidence at 15 to 34 years
(B) fever and night sweats can be presenting symptoms of Hodgkin's disease
(C) eosinophilia can be an associated finding
(D) in most patients with Hodgkin's disease, the initial mode of spread occurs via lymphatic channels to contiguous lymph nodes
(E) staging laparotomy is mandatory in every patient with Hodgkin's disease

409. All of the following statements regarding Burkitt's lymphoma are true EXCEPT that

(A) Burkitt's lymphoma is the most common form of lymphoma in children in the United States
(B) Burkitt's lymphoma in Africa is almost always associated with Epstein-Barr virus (EBV)
(C) translocation of chromatin from chromosome 8 to 14 (t8;14) is a common cytogenetic abnormality
(D) Burkitt's lymphoma is a form of B-cell lymphoma
(E) with modern aggressive combination chemotherapy over 50 percent of patients with Burkitt's lymphoma can be expected to have prolonged survival

410. All of the following statements regarding medulloblastoma are true EXCEPT that

(A) the incidence of medulloblastoma is increased in individuals with the basal cell nevus syndrome
(B) the most common location of medulloblastoma in children is in one of the cerebellar hemispheres
(C) medulloblastoma frequently metastasizes along the pathway of the cerebrospinal fluid (CSF)
(D) medulloblastoma is usually a radiosensitive tumor
(E) the level of polyamines in the CSF of many patients with medulloblastoma is elevated

411. All of the following statements about the treatment of childhood acute lymphoblastic leukemia are true EXCEPT that

(A) the use of vincristine and prednisone can produce remission in 80 to 90 percent of patients
(B) patients who fail to achieve remission after four weeks of induction therapy have a poor prognosis
(C) effective presymptomatic treatment of the central nervous system after remission induction has resulted in a decrease in the incidence of meningeal relapse from over 50 percent to less than 10 percent
(D) patients who relapse in the bone marrow while on treatment can still achieve remission in 90 percent of cases but the remission is usually short lived
(E) approximately 50 percent of patients relapse after discontinuation of therapy

412. The polymorphonuclear neutrophil shown in the illustration below is most likely to be associated with

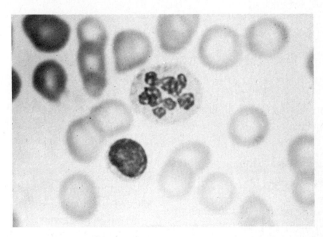

(A) malignancy
(B) iron deficiency
(C) folic acid deficiency
(D) Dohle's inclusion bodies
(E) the Pelger-Huët nuclear anomaly

413. All of the following therapies would constitute a suitable treatment of choice for at least one of the following anemias — acquired aplastic anemia, Fanconi's anemia, congenital hypoplastic anemia, or transient erythroblastopenia of childhood — EXCEPT

(A) doing nothing
(B) performing bone marrow transplantation from HLA-matched donor
(C) administering prednisone
(D) administering androgens (oxymetholene)
(E) administering glutathione

DIRECTIONS: Each question below contains four suggested answers of which **one or more** is correct. Choose the answer:

A	if	**1, 2, and 3**	are correct
B	if	**1 and 3**	are correct
C	if	**2 and 4**	are correct
D	if	**4**	is correct
E	if	**1, 2, 3, and 4**	are correct

414. Correct statements about osteosarcoma include which of the following?

(1) Osteosarcoma is rare in preschool children, but its incidence sharply rises during adolescence
(2) About 50 percent of osteosarcomas occur in the area of the knee (distal femur or proximal tibia or fibula)
(3) The most common sites of metastasis are the lungs and pleura
(4) The role of current adjuvant chemotherapy after ablative surgery in improving cure rate is well defined

415. Factors within the spleen that may adversely affect red blood cell metabolism include

(1) glucose deprivation
(2) acidic pH
(3) hypoxia
(4) high microsomal heme oxygenase activity

416. A young primigravid woman gives birth to a male infant after an uneventful full-term pregancy and a prolonged vertex delivery. Except for ecchymoses of the occipital area and a few purpuric spots over the shoulder and chest, the infant appears to be well. His platelet count is 30,000/mm³; all other tests are normal. The mother's platelet count is normal and serologic examination is negative for antiplatelet antibodies. On the third day after birth, the child appears mildly jaundiced, lethargic, and jittery, and he refuses his feedings.

At this point, ideal management of the child's thrombocytopenia would include

(1) partial excision of the spleen
(2) exchange transfusion using fresh whole blood
(3) administration of corticosteroids
(4) transfusion of washed maternal platelets

417. Poor prognostic signs in children who have acute lymphocytic leukemia include which of the following?

(1) Age below two years or above ten years
(2) Median white blood cell count at diagnosis of 20,000/mm³ or more
(3) Presence of mediastinal mass
(4) Early central nervous system leukemia

418. Von Willebrand's disease can be associated with which of the following pathologic states?

(1) Concordant decrease in the levels of antihemophilic factor (factor VIII AHF) and factor VIII antigen (factor VIII AGN)
(2) Abnormal platelet aggregation by collagen, adenosine diphosphate, and epinephrine in most patients
(3) Abnormal ristocetin-induced platelet aggregation in most patients
(4) Frequency of hemarthrosis equal to that in classical hemophilia A

---

419. A two-year-old child in shock has fulminant meningococcemia; petechiae are noted and oozing from puncture sites has been observed. The child's peripheral blood smear, presented below, shows fragmented red blood cells and few platelets. Clotting studies are likely to show

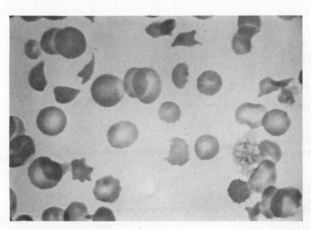

(1) decreased levels of factors V and VIII
(2) a decreased prothrombin level
(3) a decreased fibrinogen level
(4) the presence of fibrin split products

420. Hypochromic anemia is likely to be associated with which of the following disorders?

(1) Iron deficiency
(2) Anemia due to lead intoxication
(3) Thalassemia
(4) Pyridoxine-responsive anemia

421. The splenectomy of a two-year-old child has been recommended. In regard to the child's chances of developing an overwhelming infection after surgery it is true that

(1) institution of high-dose penicillin therapy for febrile illnesses can reduce the chances
(2) the salvaging of at least part of the spleen, if possible, can reduce the chances
(3) immunization with pneumococcal polysaccharide (PPS) vaccine can reduce the chances
(4) the chances are higher in this child than in a splenectomized four-year-old child

422. A 22-year-old Rh-negative primigravid woman (at 12 weeks gestation) went to a prenatal clinic after a two-day episode of spotting of blood. Indirect antiglobulin screening, which was negative at four weeks gestation, again was negative, and the woman returned home. The rest of the pregnancy was uneventful (indirect antiglobulin screening at 28 weeks was negative). Delivery was spontaneous with slight antepartum hemorrhage, and she gave birth to a healthy Rh-positive ABO-compatible infant who had no evidence of hemolytic disease. The woman received a single 300 μg prophylactic dose of Rh-immune globulin within 72 hours of delivery. Six months postpartum, however, she showed evidence of Rh sensitization, and her next pregnancy ended in the delivery of an infant who had moderately severe erythrobastosis fetalis.

Which of the following factors could have contributed to the apparent failure of Rh-immune globulin protection in this case?

(1) The woman was not monitored adequately during pregnancy
(2) The woman suffered a threatened abortion at 12 weeks and should have received a dose of Rh-immune globulin then
(3) Rh isoimmunization could have occurred between the 38th gestational week and the time of delivery
(4) Massive transplacental fetomaternal hemorrhage warranting more than a single prophylactic dose of Rh-immune globulin could have occurred

423. The overall prevalence of iron deficiency anemia in American children between the ages of six months and two years has remained stable during the last three decades despite the increasing availability of iron-fortified foods. True statements regarding preventive measures against iron deficiency anemia include which of the following?

(1) Breast milk is a better source of iron than cow's milk
(2) Cow's milk is a better source of iron than commercial formulas
(3) Iron supplementation for premature infants should begin at two months of age
(4) The best commercial cereals are those containing sodium iron pyrophosphate

424. Incidental factors affecting hemoglobin concentration and hematocrit values in a normal newborn infant include

(1) the site of blood sampling
(2) previous fetomaternal blood exchange
(3) the length of time between birth and blood sampling
(4) the manner in which the umbilical cord is clamped at the time of delivery

425. Because of fetal distress, labor is induced at 41 weeks gestation in a 40-year-old diabetic mother who has moderate toxemia of pregnancy. Induction of labor leads to the spontaneous delivery of an infant who on examination is small for gestational age, looks plethoric, and is in mild respiratory distress. Signs of Down's syndrome also are present. Laboratory data include a venous hemoglobin concentration of 26 g/100 ml and a venous hematocrit of 75%.

The polycythemia in this newborn may be attributable to

(1) maternal diabetes
(2) placental insufficiency
(3) maternal-fetal transfusion
(4) Down's syndrome

426. Assay of serum ferritin is a new tool in evaluating iron nutrition. Its advantages over the traditional measurements of hemoglobin, hematocrit, and serum transferrin saturation include which of the following?

(1) It allows evaluation of iron status within the normal range as well as in deficiency and excess
(2) Return of serum ferritin to normal levels reflects the effect of iron supplementation more reliably than do such returns of hemotocrit and transferrin saturation
(3) In anemia caused by infection or chronic disease, consistently elevated values of serum ferritin are a more reliable indicator of iron status than are values of transferrin saturation
(4) Serum ferritin is a better estimate of a mobile pool of iron than transferrin saturation

427. A preterm black male infant was found to be jaundiced 12 hours after birth. At 36 hours of age, his serum bilirubin was 18 mg/dl, hemoglobin concentration was 12.5 g/dl, and reticulocyte count 9%. Many nucleated red cells and some spherocytes were seen in the peripheral blood smear. The differential diagnosis should include

(1) glucose-6-phosphate dehydrogenase deficiency
(2) hereditary spherocytosis
(3) ABO incompatibility
(4) Rh incompatibility

DIRECTIONS: The groups of questions below consist of lettered choices followed by several numbered items. For each numbered item select the **one** lettered choice with which it is **most** closely associated. Each lettered choice may be used once, more than once, or not at all.

Questions 428–432

For each question or disorder listed, select the peripheral blood smear below with which it is most likely to be associated.

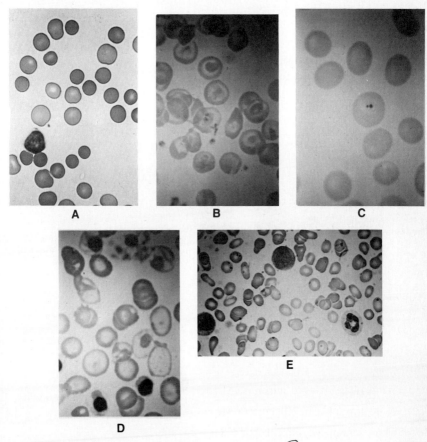

428. Howell-Jolly bodies in a splenectomized child *C*

429. Basophilic stippling in a child who has lead intoxication *D*

430. Thalassemia major *E*

431. Hereditary spherocytosis *A*

432. Hemoglobin C disease *B*

Questions 433–435

For each type of childhood leukemia listed, choose the bone marrow photomicrograph below with which it is most likely to be associated.

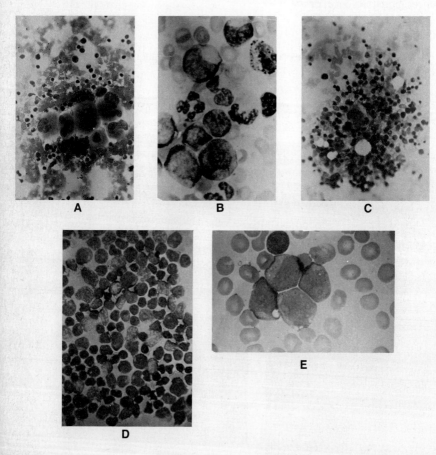

433. Acute lymphoblastic leukemia (ALL)

434. Acute myeloblastic leukemia (AML)

435. Chronic granulocytic leukemia (CGL)

Questions 436–440

Circulating hemoglobin mass reflects the balance between red blood cell production and destruction. For each of the following types of nutritional anemia, select the hematologic disorder with which it is most likely to be associated.

(A) Primarily a failure of red blood cell production often associated with increased plasma volume
(B) Primarily a failure of red blood cell production often complicated by mild to moderate red blood cell destruction
(C) Primarily red blood cell destruction that is incompletely compensated by red blood cell production
(D) Primarily red blood cell destruction accompanied by complete failure of red blood cell production (erythroid aplasia)

436. Iron deficiency anemia *B*

437. Folate deficiency anemia *B*

438. Vitamin B$_{12}$ deficiency anemia *B*

439. Vitamin E deficiency anemia *C*

440. Anemia of uncomplicated protein-calorie malnutrition *A*

Questions 441–445

Match the following chemotherapeutic agents with their corresponding mechanisms of action (as supported by cell kinetic studies).

(A) Impairs DNA synthesis by competitive inhibition of DNA polymerase
(B) Damages the microtubules in the mitotic spindle
(C) Alkylates purine bases in the DNA chain, leading to inhibition of DNA synthesis
(D) Binds to dehydrofolate reductase to prevent pyrimidine synthesis
(E) Blocks purine synthesis by inhibiting key enzymatic reactions

441. Cyclophosphamide *C*

442. 6-Mercaptopurine *E*

443. Methotrexate *D*

444. Cytosine arabinoside *A*

445. Vincristine *B*

Hematologic and Neoplastic Diseases

Answers

391.   The answer is D. *(Oski, ed 3. p 184. Cines, N Engl J Med 306:826, 1982.)* Thrombocytopenia and hemolytic anemia are common manifestations of the TORCH (toxoplasmosis, rubella, cytomegalovirus, and herpes simplex) infections as well as congenital syphilis. Both increased platelet destruction and impaired production of platelets may be the mechanism involved. Aspiration of amniotic fluid can lead to thrombocytopenia, probably because of amniotic fluid-induced platelet aggregation in the pulmonary capillary bed. Some mothers who have had ITP and who have high levels of antiplatelet antibody in the maternal plasma can give birth to thrombocytopenic infants owing to transplacental crossing of antiplatelet IgG antibody. The syndrome of congenital amegakaryocytic thrombocytopenia and bilateral absence of the radii is a well-known entity. Maternal ingestion of aspirin can lead to bleeding in the newborn, not as a result of thrombocytopenia but as a consequence of transient impairment of platelet aggregation of the infant's platelets.

392.   The answer is C. *(Nathan, ed 2. pp 726–799.)* Homozygous β-thalassemia, or Cooley's anemia, is a severe inherited anemia due to decreased synthesis of beta globin chains. Almost every patient requires frequent transfusion therapy. Each 250 ml unit of packed red blood cells contains approximately 250 mg of iron; the usual requirement of 2 units every three or four weeks will result in an excess accumulation of 50 g of iron in ten years. (The total body iron in a normal adult is 4 to 5 g.) These patients also have increased iron absorption due to excess erythropoiesis and some hypoxia due to anemia. This excess iron can damage liver, spleen, pancreas, and almost any other organ, but the worst effect is on the heart. Acute pericarditis (19 of 46 patients in one series) is a rather benign complication that has its onset at about 11 years of age. However, cardiac arrhythmias and congestive heart failure were the leading causes of death in this series (24 to 25 patients). The average age of onset was sixteen years; fourteen died within three months of onset of this complication, and only seven lived more than one year after the onset of heart failure. Autopsy findings showed severe myocardial hemosiderosis. More effective chelation therapy may postpone this inevitable complication.

393.   The answer is C. *(Nathan, ed 2. pp 838–845.)* Neutropenia in children can arise from disorders of proliferation of committed stem cells (such as cyclic neutropenia) or from disorders of proliferation of committed myeloid stem cells (such as benign neutropenia and Kostman's syndrome). Neutropenia can also be associated with abnormalities of the T and B lymphocytes, phenotypic abnormalities (such as Shwachman-Diamond syndrome and cartilage-hair hypoplasia), bone marrow replacement (e.g., leukemia or lymphoma), vitamin B12 or folate deficiency, bone marrow suppression by drugs (such as sulfonamides, anticonvulsants), certain infections, immune mediated destruction of neutrophils, and hypersplenism. In this patient, the absence of a past history of serious infection makes Kostman's syndrome the least likely diagnosis because Kostman's syndrome, usually an autosomal recessive disorder, is associated with chronic severe neutropenia and severe and often lethal pyogenic infections of the skin and respiratory tract, usually beginning during the first month of life. The outcome is usually fatal in early life.

394. The answer is D. *(Lux, Pediatr Clin North Am 27:463–486, 1980. Sullivan, Pediatr Ann 9:38–42, 1980.)* During its usual life span of 120 days, the red cell not only must maintain an adequate energy supply through utilization of glucose, but it also must keep a structural integrity and deformability to be able to negotiate its passage through small capillaries (2 to 3 μm) and the mechanically and metabolically stressful environment of the spleen. In the last few years, new data about red cell structural proteins and membrane skeleton (spectrin, actin, and ankyrin) suggest the existence of a qualitative defect that renders hereditary spherocytic red cells unstable and easily fragmented. The sequence of changes which ends with red cell death begins with loss of membrane fragments, which causes a decreased surface area/volume ratio (spherocytosis), with decreased cellular deformability. This leads to splenic entrapment and red cell death. The congested, acidic, hypoglycemic environment of the splenic cords accelerates spherocyte formation in hereditary spherocytosis (HS) more than in other conditions. Because it abolishes the hemolytic process, splenectomy is almost curative in HS. The red cells take on a more uniform morphology after splenectomy. Although splenectomy may be of marginal benefit in pyruvate kinase deficiency and hexokinase deficiency, it is of no benefit in glucose-6-phosphate dehydrogenase deficiency and acquired idiopathic hemolytic anemia.

395. The answer is C. *(Williams, ed 2. pp 1151–1152.)* The clinical history and the presence of foam cells in the bone marrow of the infant described in the question are typical of Niemann-Pick disease (sphingomyelin lipidosis). A deficiency of the lysosomal enzyme sphingomyelinase in several tissues causes the accumulation of sphingomyelin, which is ingested by reticuloendothelial cells. The resulting rounded or oval cells (foam cells) have an eccentric nucleus with prominent nucleoli; however, the distinguishing characteristic is the appearance of small, glittering droplets in the cytoplasm. These abnormal cells can be found in the bone marrow, liver, spleen, lymph nodes, thymus, brain, and many other organs. The foam cells of Gaucher's disease typically look different; the cytoplasm of these Gaucher cells appears to be stuffed with many long, wavy fibrils of variable length, giving the appearance of wrinkled tissue paper.

396. The answer is C. *(Nathan, ed 2. pp 1189–1235.)* The prolongation of PT, aPTT, and TT excludes the diagnosis of ITP. PT tests principally for factors I, II, V, VII, and X and is not prolonged in hemophilia A (factor VIII deficiency). In liver disease PT, aPTT, and TT are all prolonged, but the level of factor VIII, which is not synthesized in the liver, is normal and the platelet count is usually normal unless there is associated hypersplenism. In vitamin K deficiency there is a decrease in the production of factors II, VII, IX, and X, and PT and aPTT are prolonged. However, the thrombin time, which tests for conversion of fibrinogen to fibrin, should be normal and the platelet count should also be normal. In DIC, there is consumption of fibrinogen, factors II, V, and VIII, and platelets. Therefore, there is prolongation of PT, aPTT, and TT and decrease in factor VIII level and platelet count. In addition, the titer of fibrin split production is usually increased.

397. The answer is E. *(Halliday, Semin Hematol 19(1): 42–53, 1982.)* Deferox-amine (Desferol) is the only clinically useful iron-chelating drug in widespread usage. Theoretically, about 100 mg of deferoxamine can bind 9.35 mg of iron to the water-soluble complex in the urine. The major source of chelatable iron appears to be ferritin and hemosiderin in the storage pool of reticuloendothelial and parenchymal cells. The problem has been to accomplish effective chelation from these sites to achieve negative iron balance. Although the intramuscular route has been conventionally used for the last several years, poor solubility, painful injections, and rapid drug excretion (four to six hours) have been drawbacks. A 24-hour intravenous infusion of an equivalent dose can increase urinary iron excretion by 300 percent, but this requires hospitalization. A small lightweight infusion pump has been devised by which a 12-hour subcutaneous infusion of deferoxamine, 750 mg, can be given, increasing iron excretion by slightly over 100 percent in comparison with the same dose administered intramuscularly. This excretion is further increased by 20 to 250 percent when supplemental vitamin C is given orally to maintain a normal leukocyte vitamin C concentration. A dose of 200 mg daily is adequate. Other chelating agents still under investigation are rhodotorulic acid and 2,3-dihydrobenzoic acid.

398. The answer is D. *(Nathan, ed 2. pp 219–222.)* After reaching a critical point (venous hematocrit 60% to 65%), hyperviscosity increases exponentially, resulting in a decreased peripheral flow. The lungs, heart, and central nervous system are most affected; common symptoms and signs include respiratory distress, cyanosis, congestive heart failure, convulsions, and jaundice due to increased hemolysis. Although polycythemic patients should be monitored for evidence of hypoglycemia, hypocalcemia, and hyperbilirubinemia, in a symptomatic infant timely partial exchange transfusion using fresh frozen plasma to bring the postexchange hematocrit to 60% or below not only dramatically relieves most of the symptoms but also lessens the likelihood of future complications. The goal is to reduce the hematocrit (Hct) while maintaining the blood volume. The formula commonly employed to approximate the volume of exchange is

$$\text{Volume of exchange (ml)} = \frac{\text{blood volume} \times (\text{observed Hct} - \text{desired Hct})}{\text{observed Hct}}$$

Usually one exchange transfusion is adequate to allay the effects of a hyperviscosity problem.

399. The answer is D. *(Nathan, ed 2. pp 315–321.)* Intestinal blood loss is frequently a contributing factor in the pathogenesis of irondeficiency anemia. This blood loss almost always ceases once iron replacement treatment is started and intake of cow's milk is reduced. Blood loss also can occur due to anatomic lesions, such as Meckel's diverticula, intestinal duplications, hemorrhagic telangiectasia, or bleeding ulcers; unfortunately, these are easily overlooked in a child because of their uncommon occurrence and paucity of symptoms. Blood loss caused by these lesions must be suspected in anemic children older than two years of age or whose intestinal blood loss or anemia persists or recurs after iron treatment.

Two errors were made in the management of the patient presented in the question. First, the presence of occult blood in the stool should have been tested after the initiation of iron treatment at 18 months of age. Second and more significant, when the child was four years of age and irondeficiency anemia recurred, an immediate search for occult blood loss should have begun. A hemolytic anemia is not suggested by the data presented, and it certainly would not have responded to iron therapy.

400. The answer is D. *(Luban, Am J Pediatr Hematol/Oncol 4(1): 61–65, 1982. Karayalcin, Am J Dis Child 133: 306, 1979.)* In a longitudinal study of children with sickle cell anemia, the height and weight were found to be significantly reduced and the bone ages were significantly retarded. The Tannner staging was appropriate for bone age rather than chronological age, suggesting delayed maturation. However, the pituitary gonadotropins were found to be increased during puberty, and the thyroid and adrenal function tests were also normal, suggesting an intact pituitary-hypothalamic axis. In one series, cholelithiasis was found in 8 of 47 patients aged 2 to 18 years. Six out of the eight patients with cholelithiasis were aged 10 years or older.

401. The answer is B. *(Nathan, ed 2. pp 1202–1213.)* In recent years, with the development of concentrated plasma fractions, the management of hemophilia has shifted dramatically from physician's office, emergency room, or inpatient setting to successful home treatment programs. Prompt therapy has reduced costs, decreased morbidity, slowed the progression of hemophilic arthropathy and considerably normalized the life-style of the patient as well as of the family. Several recent studies have shown that if treatment is given as soon as the symptoms of a limp, failure to move an extremity, or a peculiar sensation in a joint are recognized, plasma levels of 5 to 10 percent factor VIII are adequate to control the simple spontaneous joint hemorrhages in severe hemophiliacs. With a delay in diagnosis or treatment the physical signs of a full-blown hemarthrosis often develop, with an immobile, red, warm, swollen, and tender joint. In such cases, much higher doses of factor VIII are required.

402. The answer is B. *(Altman, ed 2. pp 59–95.)* The main toxicities of vincristine include neuropathy (sensory, motor, autonomic, or cranial nerve), constipation, jaw pain, alopecia, and inappropriate antidiuretic hormone secretion. The major side effects of prednisone include cushingoid facies, truncal obesity, salt and water retention, hypertension, increased susceptibility to infection, gastric irritation, and osteoporosis. The toxicity of methotrexate is dependent on the dose, schedule, and route of administration. The major toxicities include gastrointestinal mucositis, bone marrow suppression, skin erythema, and hepatic dysfunction. 6-Mercaptopurine can cause nausea, vomiting, marrow suppression, and hepatic dysfunction. Adriamycin can lead to alopeica, nausea, vomiting, stomatitis, tissue necrosis (if drug extravasates), and bone marrow suppression. The dose-limiting factor is cardiotoxicity, and the risk of cardiotoxicity increases at cumulative doses of adriamycin above 550 mg/M^2.

403. The answer is C. *(Oski, Pediatr Clin North Am 27:237–252, 1980. Piomelli, Pediatrics 57:136–141, 1976.)* The last step of heme synthesis is the incorporation of iron into the protoporphyrin ring catalyzed by the enzyme heme synthetase. In iron deficiency, due to paucity of available iron, and likewise in the presence of lead, which inhibits the action of the heme synthetase, there is accumulation of protoporphyrin within the erythrocytes. Recently, a rapid, simple, inexpensive micromethod for the measurement of the erythrocyte porphyrinhemoglobin ratio (FEP:Hg) has become well established. By fingerprick, blood samples are spotted on a filter paper which can be left on the shelf for up to three months at room temperature. An inexpensive filter fluorometer is used for reading. The cost is a few cents per test, and one technician can run 200 tests each day, making the test applicable for field studies. Its major usefulness is in differentiating the three common causes of microcytic anemia: iron deficiency, β-thalassemia trait, and lead poisoning. The test results are normal in β-thalassemia trait because there is plenty of available iron and the defect is in decreased globin chain synthesis. Further, if a child with iron deficiency anemia has an intercurrent upper respiratory infection, or has already been started on iron therapy, the parameters of serum iron and transfusion saturation and ferritin may not reflect iron deficiency, whereas the FEP:Hg ratio remains high during iron therapy following the sequential senescence of microcytic red cells. The values return to normal in approximately 15 weeks. The values of FEP:Hg ratio are: less than 2.8 μg/g = normal; 3.5 to 17.0 μg/g = iron deficiency, lead poisoning, or both; and greater than 17.5 μg/g = lead poisoning or erythropoietic proto-porphyria.

404. The answer is A. *(Higby, Blood 55:2–8, 1980.)* In the selection of patients with acute leukemia for granulocyte transfusions, only with neutropenia patients (absolute neutrophil count of 500/mm^3 or less) and documented septicemia have granulocyte transfusions definitely improved the survival. With infections not accompanied by septicemia and infections caused by nonbacterial organisms (Pneumocystis carinii and fungi), the contribution of granulocyte transfusions to survival is not as well documented. In addition to the severity and the type of infection, the overall chances of recovery from neutropenia and of subsequent survival must also be taken into account in deciding whether to initiate granulocyte transfusion. About 3 to 5 percent of leukemic children are refractory to therapy, and they almost always die during induction therapy. The effective treatment involves administration of at least 10^{10} functional granulocytes per day (four transfusions per day) for seven days. In a posttransplant patient, the HLA match may be difficult due to the greater chances of immunologic reactions. Granulocyte transfusions are costly and not without the hazards of alloimmunization and the transmission of viruses.

405. The answer is D. *(Committee on Nutrition, Pediatrics, 58:765, 1976. Nathan, ed 2. American Academy of Pediatrics, pp 309–311.)* It is generally accepted that late anemia of prematurity stems from nutritional deficiencies (largely iron deficiency) caused by rapid growth and early depletion of already poor reserves. Full-term and premature newborns begin life with standard iron reserves of approximately 70 mg/kg body weight. In contrast to full-term infants whose birth weights double by five months of age and triple by one year of age, premature infants may triple their birth weights by six months of age. Early physiologic anemia of newborn infants, which is most evident between six and twelve weeks after birth, results from decreased red blood cell survival, decreased oxygen requirements, increased oxygen unloading capacity, and an absence of erythropoietin synthesis. These factors are all common in newborns but are somewhat more pronounced in premature infants. This is why iron supplementation is recommended for premature infants at two months of age.

406. The answer is E. *(D'Angio, Cancer 45:1791–1798, 1980. D'Angio, Cancer 47:2302–2311, 1981.)* The primary role of surgery (nephrectomy) is indisputable in the broad therapeutic approach to Wilms' tumor; it can confirm the diagnosis as well as contribute to clinicopathologic staging. The most significant major advance in the last decade in treating Wilms' tumor, however, has been the initiation of maintenance combination chemotherapy with actinomycin D and vincristine. The National Wilms' Tumor Study has shown that when actinomycin D or vincristine is used alone, the two-year disease-free rate is 55 percent; with combination therapy it rises to 90 percent. Similar results have been reported from Toronto and the Medical Research Council in the United Kingdom. This maintenance chemotherapy has eliminated the use of routine postoperative radiation therapy in group I disease where tumor is limited to the kidney and is completely excised. This minimizes the late consequences of radiation therapy. A third drug, adriamycin, is probably useful in some patients with more advanced disease.

407. The answer is C. *(Levine, pp 663–682.)* Neuroblastoma is a malignancy seen predominantly in the young, reflecting the congenital nature of its origin. About half of the neuroblastomas occur during the first two years of life. Neuroblastoma can arise anywhere along the course of the sympathetic nervous system. Involvement of the cervical or upper thoracic sympathetic nervous system can manifest with Horner's syndrome and/or heterochromia iridis. Two-thirds of patients, when first seen, have metastases, especially to liver, bones, bone marrow, skin, and lymph nodes. Approximately three-fourths of all tumors secrete catecholamines (vanillyl mandelic acid and homovanillic acid). Serial measurements of the urinary catecholamines have value in predicting prognosis. The two-year survival is significantly better in patients in whom the urinary catecholamine levels normalize as compared with patients in whom the levels fail to normalize or increase progressively.

408. The answer is E. *(Altman, ed 2. pp 297–329.)* In underdeveloped countries the peak incidence of Hodgkin's disease is under 10 years of age; however, in the developed countries the peak incidence occurs in late adolescence and young adulthood. There is a late peak after the age of 50. Systemic symptoms of Hodgkin's disease include fever, night sweats, malaise, weight loss, and pruritus. However, in the Ann Arbor Staging System only fever, night sweats, and weight loss are considered significant systemic symptoms that have prognostic importance. Neutrophilia occurs in about 50 percent of patients and eosinophilia in 15 to 20 percent of patients. In most instances the initial mode of spread of Hodgkin's disease is predictable involvement of contiguous lymphoid tissue. The objective of surgical staging is to determine whether there is occult intraabdominal disease in patients who clinically have only apparent supradiaphragmatic involvement. The information provided by staging laporotomy is important if radiation therapy is the only modality of treatment contemplated. In patients who have obvious intraabdominal disease by noninvasive studies (such as CAT scan or lymphangiogram) or obvious metastases outside the lymphatic system (e.g., bone marrow), combination chemotherapy with or without radiation therapy is generally recommended and staging laparotomy is then not required.

409. The answer is A. *(Levine, pp 473–574.)* Burkitt's lymphoma, a form of B-cell lymphoma, although common in equatorial Africa (100 per million children), is a very rare form of lymphoma in children in the United States (1 to 2 per million children). EBV is almost always associated with the African variety of Burkitt's lymphoma but is uncommonly connected with Burkitt's lymphoma diagnosed in the United States. t(8;14) is a very common cytogenetic abnormality in Burkitt's lymphoma. Prior to the modern combination chemotherapy era, very few children with Burkitt's lymphoma achieved prolonged survival. Current intensive chemotherapy with cyclophosphamide, adriamycin, vincristine, prednisone, and methotrexate can produce prolonged survival in over 50 percent of patients.

410. The answer is B. *(Altman, ed 2. pp 347–767.)* Primary brain tumors, such as medulloblastoma, occur with increased frequency in patients with ataxia telangiectasia, basal cell nevus syndrome, hereditary neurocutaneous disorders, and familial glioma polyposis syndrome. In children, medulloblastoma is usually a midline tumor most probably arising from the posterior medullary velum; in older adolescents and adults there is an increased incidence of medulloblastoma arising from the cerebellar hemispheres. Medulloblastomas usually spread along the pathway of the CSF and can seed many parts of the brain and spinal cord. Rarely, medulloblastoma can spread outside the nervous system to bone, bone marrow, lymph nodes, or abdominal cavity (via a ventriculoperitoneal shunt). The standard treatment is surgical resection followed by irradiation of the craniospinal axis. Trials of adjuvant chemotherapy have shown promise, and the role of chemotherapy will be better defined in the near future. The level of CSF polyamines is elevated in many patients with medulloblastoma and can be used to monitor progress of disease or to detect early recurrence.

411. The answer is E. *(Altman, ed 2. pp 239–296.)* Vincristine and prednisone are the standard drugs used in remission induction for childhood acute lymphoblastic leukemia. L-Asparaginase is usually added either during induction or during consolidation therapy. Patients who fail to achieve either complete remission on day 28, or partial remission on day 14, have a poor prognosis, even if they attain remission with subsequent therapy. The introduction of cranial irradiation with intrathecal methotrexate or intravenous intermediate dose methotrexate and intrathecal methotrexate in certain patients has reduced the incidence of meningeal relapse from over 50 percent to under 10 percent. Bone marrow relapse while on therapy signifies a very poor prognosis, although remission is still usually achievable with chemotherapy. Recent studies suggest that bone marrow transplantation may improve the survival of some of these patients. The optimal duration of therapy is still not clearly defined. Most patients have their therapy discontinued after two to three years of continuous remission. About 15 to 25 percent of patients relapse after cessation of therapy, usually within the first year.

412. The answer is C. *(Lindenbaum, Br J Haematol 44:511–513, 1980. Nathan, ed 2. pp 349–352.)* The finding of hypersegmented neutrophils (average count: > 3 lobes per cell) in the peripheral blood is one of the most useful laboratory aids in making an early diagnosis of folate deficiency. In adults put on a folate-deficient diet, serum folate levels become low in three weeks, and hypersegmented neutrophils appear in the bone marrow in five weeks and in the peripheral blood in seven weeks. It is only after 17 or 19 weeks that megaloblastic anemia develops. In a recent retrospective study of 357 patients with megaloblastic anemia, in 351 (98.3 percent) patients, the peripheral blood smear was found to have at least one hypersegmented neutrophil with six or more lobes per 100 cells. In contrast, only 1 of the 50 controls had a single six-lobed neutrophil. The Pelger-Huët anomaly is an inherited disorder in which neutrophils have no more than two lobes. Neutrophils in severe bacterial infections have toxic granulation, Dohle's inclusion bodies, and cytoplasmic vacuoles.

413. The answer is E. *(Lipton, Pediatr Clin North Am 27:217–235, 1980.)* Although uncommon, aplastic anemia is a serious childhood disease. It is strictly defined as acquired or constitutional bone marrow failure, which involves erythrocytes, granulocytes, and platelets, with peripheral pancytopenia; evidence of reduced or absent production of blood cells in the bone marrow; and replacement of normal cellular elements by fat. In a recent review of 205 pediatric patients with aplastic anemia ranging in age from newborn to 20 years of age, 30 percent had congenital or inherited types. The peak age incidence for acquired aplastic anemia was three to five years, with a poorer prognosis in the severe forms, in which the median survival was less than six months. Although there may be rare cases of spontaneous recovery or improvement, bone marrow transplantation should be performed without delay in those patients with histocompatible donors. The three-year survival rate with this procedure is approximately 50 to 70 percent, which is considerably higher than with any other therapeutic modality. Chronic graft-versus-host disease remains a morbid problem. Prior to the effective use of androgens, almost all patients with Fanconi's anemia died of complications of pancytopenia. With androgen therapy, 50 percent survive for more than seven years, but there are reports of malignant disease appearing in long-term survivors. Congenital hypoplastic anemia (Diamond-Blackfan syndrome) is a rare pure red blood cell aplasia which usually presents at birth. One-third of the patients may show short webbed neck and thumb abnormalities. Oral prednisone therapy induces a response within four weeks in 80 to 85 percent of children. The long-term prognosis is excellent. Transient erythroblastopenia of childhood is, as the name implies, a transient suppression of erythropoiesis following a viral infection. Spontaneous total recovery occurs without sequelae, and no treatment is required.

414. The answer is A (1,2,3). *(Levine, pp 575–602.)* Osteosarcoma is a tumor primarily of the 10- to 20-year-old age group, suggesting a correlation between the occurrence of the tumor and the rate of bone growth. It most frequently affects the metaphyses of long bones, especially the distal femur and proximal tibia or fibula. Although lungs and pleura are the most common sites of metastases, the tumor can also spread to other bones, lymph nodes, pericardium, kidneys, brain, and adrenal glands. There are controversies regarding the beneficial role of adjuvant chemotherapy after ablative surgery. Although many trials on chemotherapy have been performed, they were mostly nonrandomized studies, and the ultimate disease-free survival has been about 45 to 50 percent. Investigators at the Mayo Clinic have reported in a small randomized study that an actuarial two-year relapse-free survival of 52 percent was observed with or without adjuvant chemotherapy. A multicentered randomized study is now in progress.

415. The answer is A (1, 2, 3). *(Nathan, ed 2. pp 269–271.)* Stasis and slow circulation through the congested red pulp of the spleen bring about hypoxia, a fall in glucose content, and a fall in pH due to lactic acid formation. These factors together affect the metabolism and deformability of every red blood cell, especially those that are aged or abnormal. For example, a fall in pH can lower 2, 3-diphosphoglycerate activity in red blood cells, and a decrease in glucose concentration can affect the red blood cell glycolytic pathway. The effect of these environmental factors is a decrease in the deformability of red blood cells. Microsomal heme oxygenase is a heme-splitting enzyme that acts only when hemoglobin is released from a hemolyzed red blood cell; thus, it does not affect red blood cell metabolism or membrane function.

416. The answer is D (4). *(Oski, ed 3. pp 190–196.)* Isoimmune neonatal purpura is the most common cause of neonatal thrombocytopenia; it is associated with significant morbidity and mortality, particularly due to bleeding in the central nervous system. The pathogenesis is very similar to that of isoimmune Rh-immunization. The techniques for the determination of platelet antigens and the antibodies directed against them can be useful in diagnosis. One should also exclude idiopathic thrombocytopenic purpura in the mother and intrauterine infection and sepsis in the neonate. Platelet transfusion may be of both therapeutic and diagnostic value. Because platelets from an affected infant's mother may be associated with a significant dose of plasma antibodies, they should be washed before transfusion into the child. Isoimmune neonatal purpura is likely to recur in subsequent pregnancies; cesarean section therefore should be done in the case of a thrombocytopenic fetus in whom a fetal scalp blood sample is obtained at the onset of labor.

417. The answer is E (all). *(Mauer, Blood 56:1–10, 1980. Altman, ed 2. pp 253–256.)* Age less than two years or more than ten years, the presence at diagnosis of central nervous system leukemia or a white blood cell count of 20,000/mm³ or higher, and the appearance of a mediastinal mass all indicate a poor prognosis for children who have acute lymphocytic leukemia. Most of the children having these poor prognostic signs have the thymic (T cell) variety of the disease. These children, usuallly older boys, possess surface antigens specific for thymocytes. In addition to the conventionally employed regimen of prednisone and vincristine, other chemotherapeutic agents, such as daunorubicin or L-asparaginase, should be administered. Children with T-cell acute lymphocytic leukemia run a greater risk of bleeding and infection during the first four weeks of remission induction therapy. Only 20 percent of these patients with poor prognostic features can be expected to achieve long-term disease-free survival, and once they relapse, which is very often in the first few months, virtually none of them go into remission despite aggressive chemotherapy.

418. The answer is B (1, 3). *(Nathan, ed 2. pp 1214–1219.)* Von Willebrand's disease (VWD) usually presents as epistaxis and easy bruising in early childhood. In contrast to classical hemophilia A, hemarthrosis and fatal bleeding are unusual. Although factor VIII procoagulant activity (factor VIII AHF) is decreased in both disorders, hemophiliac plasma contains an antigen that is precipitated by a rabbit antibody to factor VIII (factor VIII AGN), whereas patients with severe VWD lack this antigen. The prolonged bleeding time in VWD is due to a defect in platelet adhesiveness as documented by significant impairment of ristocetin-induced platelet aggregation in the majority of patients. This factor, which is missing in plasma in VWD, is called von Willebrand's factor (factor VIII VWF). Platelet aggregation by collagen, adenosine diphosphate, and epinephrine is normal in most patients with VWD. These tests are used to confirm the diagnosis of VWD and to differentiate it from classical hemophilia A.

419. The answer is E (all). *(Nathan, ed 2. pp 1223–1228.)* The clinical history and blood-smear findings presented in the question are typical of disseminated intravascular coagulation. The disorder, which can be triggered by endotoxin shock, results ultimately in the initiation of the intrinsic clotting mechanism and the generation of thrombin. Fibrin deposited in the microcirculatory system can lead to tissue ischemia and necrosis, further capillary damage, release of thromboplastic substances, and increased thrombin generation. Simultaneous activation of the fibrinolytic system produces increased amounts of fibrin split products, which inhibit thrombin activity. Of utmost importance in the treatment of children who have disseminated intravascular coagulation is the management of the condition that precipitated the disorder.

420.   The answer is E (all). *(Nathan, ed 2. pp 329–332.)* Red blood cells emerging from the bone marrow with decreased amounts of hemoglobin first become smaller (microcytic) in order to sustain an adequate mean corpuscular hemoglobin concentration and only later become hypochromic and show increased central pallor on peripheral-smear examination. The impairment could be in the synthesis of globin or heme. In thalassemia, there is a quantitative decrease in globin-chain synthesis due to a genetic disorder. In iron deficiency, synthesis of heme is impaired due to lack of iron; and lead can block incompletely many enzymatic steps in heme manufacture. In pyridoxine-responsive anemia, the exact mechanism causing hypochromicity is unknown, but the impairments resemble those of lead poisoning and result in poor utilization of adequate iron stores situated in the normoblasts.

421.   The answer is E (all). *(Gellis, pp 276–278.)* The immune functions of the spleen, other than the filtration and phagocytosis of bacteria in the reticuloendothelial system, are not completely known. After splenectomy, the serum level of immunoglobulin M falls and opsonization of encapsulated organisms like *Streptococcus (Diplococcus) pneumoniae* becomes defective. These factors may contribute to the development of overwhelming pneumococcal infections in splenectomized children, especially those who are less than four years of age, who have a severe hematologic disease, or who require chemotherapy for a lymphoma. A recent follow-up evaluation of 71 splenectomized or autosplenectomized patients who were immunized with pneumococcal polysaccharide (PPS) vaccine revealed that this vaccine is effective in preventing pneumococcal sepsis. Although the use of prophylactic penicillin in splenectomized children has on occasion been recommended, it is not known for how many years prophylaxis should be continued or whether it can prevent sepsis caused by gram-negative organisms. An aggressive approach to febrile illness in children should be undertaken, including institution of high-dose penicillin therapy before blood culture results are available.

422.   The answer is E (all). *(Bowman, pp 40–47. Oski, ed 3. pp 323–326.)* The incidence of Rh immunization can be reduced from 15 percent to 2 percent by postdelivery injections of Rh-immune globulin. The case history presented illustrates several problems in reducing the failure rate of Rh prevention. Proper monitoring of this woman should have included a Kleihauer acid elution test (to demonstrate fetal cells in her circulation) at the time of the threatened abortion and also, because of antepartum hemorrhage, after delivery. Furthermore, if initial sensitization produced minimal antibody levels, more sensitive screening techniques should have been used, even after 28 weeks gestation; the usual indirect antiglobulin antibody screen alone may be negative. Thus, she should have received one dose of Rh-immune globulin at 12 weeks and more than one dose after delivery, if there was significant fetomaternal bleeding.

423. The answer is B (1, 3). *(American Academy of Pediatrics, Pediatrics 58:765–768, 1976. Dallman, p 6.)* The Committee of Nutrition of the American Academy of Pediatrics states that iron supplementation from one or two sources, such as the newer iron-fortified cereals (that do not contain the poorly absorbed iron pyrophosphate) or iron-containing drops, should begin at four months of age for term infants and two months for premature infants. Breast-feeding is preferred, and iron-fortified formulas and other heat-treated milk products are better than cow's milk as substitutes for human breast milk during the first six to twelve months of an infant's life. After the age of six months, infants receiving cow's milk should have their daily milk intake limited to 750 ml and should begin eating iron-rich solid foods. Excessive milk ingestion increases occult blood loss in the gastrointestinal tract and thus contributes to iron deficiency anemia. Unless milk drinking is discouraged and better methods of iron supplementation for infants are adopted, iron deficiency will remain all too common. It has recently been shown by using an external tagging method ($^{59}FeSO_4$) that breast-fed infants absorb 49 percent of the iron in the breast milk in contrast to infants fed cow's milk or unfortified cow's milk formula who absorbed only 10 to 12 percent of the available iron. Assessment of iron nutrition by serum ferritin measurements indicates that routine iron supplementation may not be necessary in term infants who continue to be breast-fed.

424. The answer is E (all). *(Nathan, ed 2. pp 27–31.)* Capillary blood samples from a heel prick have hemoglobin values 10 percent higher than venous samples. This error can be minimized by warming the area, eliciting a brisk blood flow, and discarding the initial drops. Within the first few hours after birth, plasma volume decreases and hemoglobin concentration increases (from 15 to 25 percent). The placental vessels at birth contain 75 to 125 ml of blood, about a quarter of which normally gets into a newborn infant within 15 seconds of birth. Cord-related factors can make a difference of 40 percent of neonatal blood volume; for example, because the umbilical arteries constrict shortly after birth, whereas the vein remains dilated, delayed cord clamping was associated in one study with an average red blood cell mass of 49 ml/kg at 72 hours as compared to 31 ml/kg in infants with immediate cord clamping. Fetomaternal transfusion in the last phases of pregnancy and labor can lead to anemia in the newborn; conversely, maternal-fetal transfusion can result in plethora.

425. The answer is E (all). *(Nathan, ed 2. pp 1509–1510.)* Polycythemia (hemoglobin, > 22 g/100 ml; hematocrit, > 65%) in an infant during the first week of life can lead to several undesirable complications. Although the etiology may be obscure, placental insufficiency leading to intrauterine hypoxia seems to play a central role in the majority of the conditions associated with plethora. Maternal diabetes, another common cause, may be related to placental dysfunction. In infants who have Down's syndrome, evidence of a myeloproliferative disorder is not uncommon; it can affect in the neonatal period any of the formed blood elements and very often is associated with myeloid hyperplasia that can be confused with congenital leukemia.

426. The answer is A (1, 2, 3). *(Nathan, ed 2. pp 217–218.)* Serum ferritin concentration is a very sensitive reflection of iron stores from birth to adult life. Its assay requires less than 0.1 ml of serum, and because samples can be stored for several months, it is a useful tool in nutritional surveys. The normal value in children between the ages of 6 months and 15 years is 30 ng/ml; the level in children who have iron deficiency anemia is 10.0 ng/ml. In iron overload (sickle cell disease) levels may be over 500 ng/ml. In the natural sequence of stages in iron deficiency, depletion of *iron stores,* as manifested by a fall in serum ferritin concentration, is the first readily detectable event. This is then followed by a fall in serum transferrin saturation (which represents the *mobile iron pool*). Only when transferrin saturation drops below 15 percent does the marrow feel the pinch of iron deficiency. Anemia is a late nonspecific manifestation of iron deficiency; in fact, iron deficiency, as reflected first by decreased ferritin levels and then by transferrin saturation, may exist for several weeks before there are clinical manifestations of anemia. Infection and chronic disease may cause transferrin synthesis but not serum ferritin concentration to drop, thus making transferrin saturation a less reliable laboratory index than serum ferritin under these conditions. Some investigators reported measuring serum ferritin in assessment of iron nutrition in 238 infants on seven occasions in the first year of life. The values of iron-supplemented infants remained consistently higher.

427. The answer is A (1,2,3). *(Oski, ed 3. pp 112–182.)* Spherocytosis can be seen in hereditary spherocytosis, G-6-PD deficiency, or ABO incompatibility. Hyperbilirubinemia has been associated with black preterm infants with G-6-PD deficiency but not with black term infants. The blood smear of the affected infant usually reveals nucleated red cells, spherocytes, poikilocytes, "blister" cells, and fragmented cells. Neonatal hyperbilirubinemia occurs in about 50 percent of patients with hereditary spherocytosis. Spherocytosis occurs in ABO incompatibility but not in Rh incompatibility. The hemolytic manifestations of ABO incompatibility and hereditary spherocytosis are very similar. One should determine the blood types of the mother and of the infant, the results of a direct Coombs' test on the infant, and the presence or absence of a family history of hemolytic disease (spherocytosis).

428–432. The answers are: 428-C, 429-E, 430-D, 431-A, 432-B. *(Nathan ed 2. pp 277, 296, 396–404, 492–502, 731–734.)* Howell-Jolly bodies (slide C) are small, spherical nuclear remnants seen in the reticulocytes and, rarely, etythrocytes of individuals who have no spleen—either due to congenital asplenia or splenectomy — or who have a poorly functioning spleen (e.g., hyposplenism associated with sickle cell disease). Ultrafiltration of blood is a unique function of the spleen that cannot be assumed by other reticuloendothelial organs.

Basophilic stippling (slide E) represents abnormal aggregates of ribosomes with reticulocytes. This condition occurs whenever the utilization of iron for hemoglobin synthesis is impeded, as in lead intoxication and thalassemia. The presented peripheral blood smear of a child who has lead poisoning also provides evidence (microcytic, hypochromic red blood cells) of associated iron deficiency.

A target cell is an erythrocyte with a membrane that is too large for its hemoglobin content; a thin rim of hemoglobin at the cell's periphery and a small disc in the center give the cell a target-like appearance. Target cells, which are more resistant to osmotic fragility than other erythrocytes, are seen in children who have β-thalassemia, hemoglobin C disease, or liver disease (e.g., obstructive jaundice or cirrhosis). Thalassemia major (slide D) can be diagnosed by the presence of poorly hemoglobinized normoblasts in addition to target cells in the peripheral blood.

Uniformly small microspherocytes (less than 6 μm in diameter) are typical of hereditary spherocytosis (slide A). Because of a decreased surface-to-volume ratio, these osmotically fragile red blood cells have an increased density of hemoglobin. Although spherical red blood cells also may appear in other hemolytic states, such as immune hemolytic anemia, microangiopathy, ABO incompatibility, and hypersplenism, their cellular volume is only irregularly augmented.

Although hemoglobin C disease (slide B) is a mild disorder, target cells comprise a far greater percentage of total red blood cells than in thalassemia major. Target cells are the only manifestations of hemoglobin C disease; targeting is so striking because hemoglobin C has a greater tendency than normal hemoglobin to aggregate and precipitate during the drying of cells on a glass slide.

433–435. The answers are: 433-D, 434-E, 435-B. *(Nathan, ed 2. pp 979–984.)* The differentiation of the types of leukemia is based mainly on morphologic characteristics as revealed by Wright's-stained smears of peripheral blood and bone marrow. Only occassionally are special cytochemical stains helpful in confirming the diagnosis.

Acute lymphoblastic leukemia is the most common type of childhood leukemia and is associated with the best prognosis. The marrow is filled with one kind of cell; most of the volume of this cell is occupied by an immature nucleus, which includes chromatin clumped around a few nucleoli. There may be folding of the nucleus. The scanty cytoplasm is blue and nongranular. Periodic acid-Schiff stain may be positive.

Acute myeloblastic leukemia is less common and has a poorer prognosis. The myeloblasts are mostly in one phase of maturity and show thin, spongy nuclear chromatin and several distinct punched-out nucleoli. The blue-gray cytoplasm is more abundant than in lymphoblasts and often contains typical Auer rods, which are abnormal lysosomes never seen in lymphoblasts. Myeloperoxidase stain may be positive.

Chronic granulocytic leukemia progresses through two stages: chronic and blastic. Bone marrow examination during the chronic phase reveals a proliferation of granulocytic cells of intermediate maturity; increased platelets also may be noted. The blastic phase, which is much harder to treat, is characterized by an increased number of less differentiated blast cells.

436–440. The answers are: 436-B, 437-B, 438-B, 439-C, 440-A. *(Nathan, ed 2. pp 289–298.)* One of the best clinical approaches in the evaluation of anemia is the determination of the status of red blood cell production and destruction. Destruction reflects a decrease in the life span of red blood cells, as evidenced by hemolysis or blood loss. The bone marrow's response to anemia is reflected by the reticulocyte count or by the presence of polychromasia in the peripheral smear. In deficiencies of iron, folate, or vitamin B_{12}, the marrow responds with increased cellularity of erythroid precursors; due to a lack of substrate, however, not enough mature red blood cells are released, and the reticulocyte count decreases. All three of these deficiencies, particularly in the advanced stages, are further complicated by red blood cell destruction both in the marrow and the peripheral blood.

In the anemia of protein-calorie malnutrition, which is due to a lack of essential amino-acid substrates, the bone marrow shows a decreased erythroid-to-myeloid ratio and a reduced population of reticulocytes. Red blood cell survival is normal. If uncomplicated (i.e., if there is no significant iron or folate deficiency due to regional environmental factors), the anemia is moderate; however, plasma volume is increased disproportionately due to hypoalbuminemia.

In premature infants, vitamin E deficiency can lead to hemolytic anemia. Because one of the metabolic roles of vitamin E compounds is to protect lipids in biologic membranes from oxidative damage, injury to red blood cell membranes can occur in vitamin E-deficient infants. Red blood cell survival is moderately decreased; and although red blood cell production is increased (reticulocyte counts usually are 10 percent), it fails to compensate completely.

441–445. The answers are: 441-C, 442-E, 443-D, 444-A, 445-B. *(Altman, ed 2. pp 59–95.)* Because experimental data concerning the use of chemotherapeutic agents are incomplete and at times, perhaps, inaccurate, much of cancer chemotherapy still is given on an empirical basis. However, since the introduction of tritiated thymidine, accurate studies of DNA synthetic activities and of the proliferative characteristics of normal and leukemic cells now are possible, and a reasonably good correlaton between in vivo and in vitro studies of leukemic cells has emerged. Several treatment advances, such as multimodal therapy using cytosine arabinoside in the treatment of children who have acute myelogenous leukemia, have resulted from these more sophisticated scientific studies.

The five antineoplastic drugs listed in the question all have different mechanisms of action. *Methotrexate* is a folic acid analog that binds in a "pseudoreversible" reaction with the enzyme dehydrofolate reductase, which is essential for the synthesis of pyrimidines. *Cytosine arabinoside* (cytarabine, ara-C) is a pyrimidine analog that impairs DNA synthesis by competitive inhibition of DNA polymerase. Both of these agents exert their antimetabolic effects during the S phase of the mitotic cycle.

Cyclophosphamide is a nitrogen mustard alkylating agent that inhibits DNA synthesis by the alkylation of purine basis. It blocks the mitotic cycle at the premitotic (G_2) stage. *Vincristine* is a vinca alkaloid, derived from the periwinkle plant; by damaging the microtubules necessary for the formation of mitotic spindles, this chemotherapeutic agent arrests mitosis during metaphase. The purine analog *6-mercaptopurine* is an effective antineoplastic drug because it blocks purine synthesis by inhibiting two enzymatic reactions: the conversion of 5-phosphoribosyl-1-pyrophosphate to 5-phosphoribosyl-1-amine and the conversion of inosinic acid to xanthylic acid.

Endocrine, Metabolic, and Genetic Disorders

Abdollah Sadeghi-Nejad

DIRECTIONS: Each question below contains five suggested answers. Choose the **one best** response to each question.

446. All of the following are among the features of the syndrome of inappropriate secretion of antidiuretic hormone (SIADH) EXCEPT

(A) hypervolemia
(B) plasma hypoosmolality
(C) inappropriately low urinary sodium (relative to serum)
(D) hyponatremia
(E) urinary hypertonicity (relative to plasma)

447. All of the following disorders are associated with neonatal hypo—glycemia EXCEPT

(A) von Gierke's disease (glucose-6-phosphatase deficiency)
(B) Pompe's disease (acid maltase deficiency)
(C) panhypopituitarism
(D) prematurity
(E) nesidioblastosis

448. Individuals who have a 48,XXXY karyotype are tall, mentally retarded phenotypic males having a small phallus and small, abnormal testes. Cells obtained by buccal smear would be expected to contain how many Barr bodies?

(A) One
(B) Two
(C) Three
(D) Four
(E) None

449. All of the following statements about neonatal thyrotoxicosis are true EXCEPT that

(A) it occurs equally in male and female infants
(B) it is thought to be caused by cross-placental passage of maternal thyroid-stimulating immunoglobulins (TSI)
(C) it is usually a self-limited disorder
(D) it could be life threatening and may require prompt, vigorous treatment
(E) it does not occur when the mother is being treated with antithyroid drugs

450. In the evaluation of thyroid function, the tests most frequently used are total serum thyroxine and T_3 resin uptake. The test T_3 uptake indirectly measures the concentration of

(A) total T_3
(B) free T_3
(C) reverse T_3
(D) free T_4
(E) thyroxine-binding globulin

451. True sexual precocity in girls is most likely to be caused by

(A) a feminizing ovarian tumor
(B) a gonadotropin-producing tumor
(C) a lesion of the central nervous system
(D) exogenous estrogens
(E) early onset of "normal" puberty (constitutional)

452. A ten-year-old obese boy is diagnosed as having Cushing's syndrome on the basis of his fat distribution, his arrested growth, and the presence of hypertension, plethora, purple striae, and osteoporosis. Which of the following disorders is most likely to be responsible for the clinical picture that this boy presents?

(A) Bilateral adrenal hyperplasia
(B) Adrenal adenoma
(C) Adrenal carcinoma
(D) Craniopharyngioma
(E) Ectopic adrenocorticotropin-producing tumor

453. According to Greek mythology, Hermaphroditus was the son of Hermes and Aphrodite. As a youth, he rejected the love of Salmacis, a river nymph. The gods granted both her wish to remain with him always and his wish to die rather than submit to her love by fusing them into one ambisexual being as they drowned in a river. All of the following statements about true hermaphrodites are true EXCEPT that

(A) most are chromatin-positive
(B) most have parents with sex-chromosome aberrations
(C) their sex-chromosome patterns may be XX, XY, or a mosaic
(D) their internal genitalia reflect the composition of their gonads
(E) they may have both a testis and an ovary

454. In many parts of the world mass screening for congenital hypothyroidism is done routinely. All of the following statements are true for this disorder EXCEPT that

(A) thyroid binding globulin (TBG) level is usually normal
(B) serum thyroxine (T_4) level is low
(C) clinical features of cretinism are usually apparent during the first weeks of life
(D) T_3 resin uptake is low
(E) Thyroid-stimulating hormone levels (TSH) may be high, normal, or low

455. A 12-year-old girl has a mass in her neck. Physical examination reveals a thyroid nodule, but the rest of the gland is not palpable. A technetium scan reveals a "cold" nodule. The child appears to be euthyroid. Which of the following diagnoses is the LEAST likely?

(A) Simple adenoma
(B) Follicular carcinoma
(C) Papillary carcinoma
(D) A cyst
(E) Dysgenetic thyroid gland

456. Regarding congenital adrenal hyperplasia (adrenogenital syndrome) caused by a deficiency of 21-hydroxylase, all of the following statements are true EXCEPT that

(A) female infants may be virilized
(B) skin hyperpigmentation may be present
(C) infants may present with hyponatremia and hyperkalemia
(D) male infants may have ambiguous genitalia
(E) it is an autosomal recessive disorder

457. Patients with pseudohypoparathyroidism are expected to have all of the following features EXCEPT

(A) hypocalcemia
(B) hyperphosphatemia
(C) elevated concentrations of parathyroid hormone
(D) shortness of stature
(E) rise in urinary phosphate excretion in response to the infusion of parathyroid hormone

458. Glycosylated hemoglobin (hemoglobin A1C) is often used as an indicator of control in patients with diabetes mellitus. Its level usually reflects the blood concentration of glucose over the preceding

(A) one month
(B) two months
(C) one week
(D) four months
(E) eight hours

459. A six-year-old girl has been referred to an endocrinologist because a reducing substance was found in her urine during a routine examination. Physical examination and glucose tolerance test results are normal; her urine reacts with Clinitest tablets but not with Clinistix. The most likely diagnosis is

(A) diabetes mellitus
(B) renal glycosuria
(C) hereditary fructose intolerance
(D) essential fructosuria
(E) deficiency of fructose-1,6-diphosphatase activity

460. A seven-day-old boy is admitted to a hospital for evaluation of vomiting and dehydration. Physical examination is normal except for minimal hyperpigmentation of the nipples. Serum sodium and potassium concentrations are 120 meq/L and 9 meq/L, respectively. The most likely diagnosis is

(A) pyloric stenosis
(B) congenital adrenal hyperplasia
(C) secondary hypothyroidism
(D) panhypopituitarism
(E) hyperaldosteronism

461. An infant is brought to a hospital because her wet diapers turn black when they are exposed to air. Physical examination is normal. Urine is positive both for reducing substance and when tested with ferric chloride. This disorder is caused by a deficiency of

(A) homogentisic acid oxidase
(B) phenylalanine hydroxylase
(C) L-histidine ammonia-lyase
(D) ketoacid decarboxylase
(E) isovaleryl-CoA dehydrogenase

462. Hereditary disorders transmitted as an X-linked recessive trait would be best described by which of the following statements?

(A) Females are not affected
(B) Heterozygous females are less severely affected than hemizygous males
(C) Hemizygous males are not affected
(D) Hemizygous males are less severely affected than heterozygous females
(E) Hemizygous males and heterozygous females are affected with equal frequency

463. Which of the following laboratory findings is unusual in patients with simple (nutritional) rickets?

(A) Aminoaciduria
(B) Hyperphosphaturia
(C) Elevated serum alkaline phosphatase levels
(D) Hypercalciuria
(E) Hypophosphatemia

464. Mental retardation of varying severity may be associated with tall stature in all of the syndromes listed below EXCEPT

(A) cerebral gigantism (Sotos' syndrome)
(B) homocystinuria
(C) XXY (Kleinfelter's syndrome)
(D) Marfan's syndrome
(E) XYY

465. Hirsutism in a phenotypic female may be caused by any of the following disorders EXCEPT

(A) congenital adrenal hyperplasia (adrenogenital syndrome)
(B) Cushing's syndrome
(C) androgen-producing ovarian tumor
(D) testicular feminization — phenotypic female with intraabdominal testes and 46,XY karyotype
(E) administration of exogenous androgens

466. Maple syrup urine disease (classical branched-chain ketoaciduria) is a hereditary disorder transmitted as an autosomal recessive trait. If the gene frequency for heterozygosity is 1 in 250, the expected incidence of the disease would be

(A) 1 in 1000
(B) 1 in 25,000
(C) 1 in 62,500
(D) 1 in 250,000
(E) 1 in 625,000

467. Neonatal hypoglycemia is common in premature and small-for-gestational-age infants. The most common cause of hypoglycemia in these infants is

(A) inadequate stores of nutrients
(B) adrenal immaturity
(C) pituitary immaturity
(D) insulin excess
(E) glucagon deficiency

468. All of the following statements about Wilson's disease are true EXCEPT that

(A) it is inherited as a sex-linked trait
(B) in children, it may present with hepatomegaly and liver failure
(C) ceruloplasmin levels are typically decreased
(D) total serum copper concentration is usually low
(E) it is often associated with renal disease (Fanconi syndrome)

469. A one-day-old infant develops tetany and convulsions. Serum calcium is 6.2 mg/100 ml. Which of the following diagnoses is the LEAST likely in this infant?

(A) Perinatal asphyxia
(B) High phosphorus intake
(C) Maternal diabetes mellitus
(D) Maternal hyperparathyroidism
(E) Prematurity

DIRECTIONS: Each question below contains four suggested answers of which **one or more** is correct. Choose the answer:

A	if	**1, 2, and 3**	are correct
B	if	**1 and 3**	are correct
C	if	**2 and 4**	are correct
D	if	**4**	is correct
E	if	**1, 2, 3, and 4**	are correct

470. Juxtaglomerular hyperplasia (Bartter's syndrome) is characterized by which of the following conditions?

(1) Hypokalemia
(2) Hyperaldosteronism
(3) Hyperreninemia
(4) Hypertension

471. Cholecalciferol (vitamin D_3) is absorbed by the gut. In its enzymatic conversion to the active form of the vitamin, it must undergo

(1) hydroxylation at carbon 25
(2) hydroxylation at carbon 24
(3) hydroxylation at carbon 1
(4) hydroxylation at carbon 3

472. Patients with the syndrome of testicular feminization are correctly described by which of the following statements?

(1) They are genotypic females
(2) Their breasts develop at puberty
(3) Their menses can be normal
(4) They exhibit end-organ resistance to testosterone

473. Hirsutism in females may be caused by

(1) increased ovarian androgens
(2) genetic predisposition
(3) increased adrenal androgens
(4) increased testicular (ectopic) androgens

474. Known causes of primary or secondary amenorrhea include

(1) hyperprolactinemia
(2) hypothyroidism
(3) hypogonadotropic hypogonadism
(4) hyperthyroidism

475. Ketonuria usually accompanies fasting in normal children. Other true statements regarding fasting in children include which of the following?

(1) Lipolysis is enhanced
(2) Blood glucose concentration frequently decreases during 24 hours of fasting
(3) Serum fatty acid levels are high
(4) Hyperinsulinemia is present

476. The best screening for growth hormone deficiency are fasting concentration of growth hormone after exercise and after treatment with estrogens. The "definitive" tests usually used include the response of growth hormone to

(1) insulin-induced hypoglycemia
(2) L-dopa
(3) arginine infusion
(4) medroxyprogesterone acetate

477. Tall stature can be a feature of which of the following conditions?

(1) Familial tall stature
(2) Congenital adrenal hyperplasia (prepubertally)
(3) Marfan's syndrome
(4) Homocystinuria

478. Known causes of hyperlacticacidemia include which of the following?

(1) Pyruvate carboxylase deficiency
(2) Pyruvate dehydrogenase deficiency
(3) Fructose-1,6-diphosphatase deficiency
(4) Phosphofructokinase deficiency

479. Physical examination of a three-year-old infant suspected of having hypothyroidism is entirely normal. Routine newborn screening of the cord blood showed a low level of thyroxine and normal concentration of thyroid-stimulating hormone. These results were confirmed two weeks later on a venous blood sample. The differential diagnosis should include

(1) thyroid-binding globulin deficiency
(2) tertiary (hypothalamic) hypothyroidism
(3) secondary (pituitary) hypothyroidism
(4) primary hypothyroidism

480. An infant girl who has a 46,XX karyotype is hospitalized to determine the cause of her ambiguous genitalia. This child's virilization is likely to be caused by

(1) maternal exposure to progestins
(2) maternal androgen intake
(3) congenital adrenal hyperplasia
(4) neonatal Cushing's syndrome

481. Goitrous hypothyroidism can be present in a newborn infant as the result of which of the following factors?

(1) Peroxidase deficiency
(2) Maternal ingestion of thyroid hormone
(3) Maternal ingestion of iodide
(4) Thyroid-stimulating hormone deficiency

482. A six-year-old boy with a two-week history of polyuria, polydipsia, and anorexia is admitted to a hospital. Which of the following diagnoses are likely?

(1) Insulin-dependent diabetes mellitus
(2) Nephrogenic diabetes insipidus
(3) Central diabetes insipidus
(4) Phosphate diabetes

DIRECTIONS: The groups of questions below consist of lettered choices followed by several numbered items. For each numbered item select the **one** lettered choice with which it is **most** closely associated. Each lettered choice may be used once, more than once, or not at all.

Questions 483–487

For each of the disorders listed below, select the serum concentration of calcium (Ca) and phosphate (PO_4) with which it is most likely to be associated.

(A) Low PO_4, normal Ca
(B) Low PO_4, high Ca
(C) Normal PO_4, low Ca
(D) Normal PO_4, normal Ca
(E) High PO_4, low Ca

483. Vitamin D-resistant rickets

484. Pseudohypoparathyroidism

485. Osteogenesis imperfecta

486. Hyperparathyroidism

487. Medullary thyroid carcinoma (primary hypercalcitoninemia)

Questions 488–493

All of the syndromes listed below are associated with obesity in children. For each of the other clinical findings that follow, select the syndrome with which it is most likely to be associated.

(A) Prader-Willi syndrome
(B) Laurence-Moon-Biedl syndrome
(C) Cushing's syndrome
(D) Frohlich's syndrome
(E) Pseudohypoparathyroidism

488. Cataracts

489. Hypotonia

490. Polydactyly

491. Brachydactyly

492. Basal ganglia calcification

493. Retinitis pigmentosa

Questions 494–500

For each of the following disorders, select the serum concentrations (meq/L) of sodium (Na$^+$) and potassium (K$^+$) with which it is most likely to be associated.

(A) Na$^+$ 118, K$^+$ 7.5
(B) Na$^+$ 120, K$^+$ 3.0
(C) Na$^+$ 134, K$^+$ 6.0
(D) Na$^+$ 144, K$^+$ 2.9
(E) Na$^+$ 155, K$^+$ 5.5

494. Salt-losing 21-hydroxylase deficiency (adrenogential syndrome)

495. Central diabetes insipidus

496. Nephrogenic diabetes insipidus

497. Hyperaldosteronism

498. Syndrome of inappropriate antidiuretic hormone (ADH) secretion

499. Addison's disease (in crisis)

500. Glucose-6-phosphatase deficiency (von Gierke's disease)

Endocrine, Metabolic, and Genetic Disorders

Answers

446. The answer is C. *(Hung, pp 110–111.)* In SIADH there is continued secretion of antidiuretic hormone despite hyponatremia, hypotonicity, and volume expansion. Thus, the urine is inappropriately concentrated and has high concentrations of sodium relative to the serum sodium concentration. The symptoms are those of water intoxication. In the pediatric patient the syndrome is usually produced when large amounts of fluids are administered intravenously to a patient who has hypersecretion of ADH in response to a disease process (such as central nervous system infections, neurosurgical procedures, or pulmonary disease). Increased ADH secretion may also be secondary to the administration of various drugs, such as some anesthetics and anticonvulsants.

448. The answer is B. *(Williams, ed 6. p 430–431.)* A Barr (chromatin) body represents a partially inactivated X chromosome. The number of Barr bodies in each cell nucleus is equal to the number of X chromosomes minus one. Thus, normal males (XY) and females who have Turner's syndrome (XO) have no Barr bodies; normal females (XX) and males with Klinefelter's syndrome (XXY) have one Barr body in each cell.

449. The answer is E. *(Rudolph, ed 17. p 1535.)* Infants born to thyrotoxic mothers may be hypothyroid, euthyroid, or hyperthyroid. Neonatal thyrotoxicosis usually disappears within two to four months as the concentration of thyroid-stimulating immunoglobulins (7S gammaglobulin) diminishes. Unlike TSI, thyroid-stimulating hormone (TSH) does not cross the placenta. All forms of thyrotoxicosis are more common in females with the exception of neonatal thyrotoxicosis, which has an equal sex distribution. In severely affected infants, the disease could be fatal if not treated vigorously and promptly. Depending on the severity of the disorder, treatment with antithyroid drugs, propanolol, and digitalis may be required.

450. The answer is E. *(Gardner, ed 2. p 330. Williams, ed 6. p 153. Hung, p 128.)* The concentration of total serum thyroxine (T_4) is influenced by an individual's metabolic state and concentration of thyroxine-binding globulin (TBG). Thus, T_4 levels are high if TBG levels are high, as for example, in the newborn state, during pregnancy, or while taking oral contraceptives; conversely, T_4 levels are low in association with TBG deficiency. Because the measurement of TBG is tedious, triiodothyronine (T_3) uptake is used as an indirect measurement of TBG; uptake of T_3 and levels of TBG are inversely related. The product of T_3 uptake and total serum T_4, the free T_4 index, is used as an indicator of free (unbound) hormone which is metabolically active.

451. The answer is E. *(Gardner, ed 2. p 619. Hung, pp 78–81.)* The term "true sexual precocity" implies that gonads have matured in response to the secretion of pituitary gonadoropins and have begun secreting sex steroids, causing the development of secondary sexual characteristics. Thus, ovarian tumors and exogenous estrogens, which suppress the function of the pituitary gland, do not cause true precocious puberty. In girls, the most common form of true precocious puberty is idiopathic and is thought to be caused by early maturation of an otherwise normal hypothalamic-pituitary-gonadal feedback system. In boys, true precocious puberty is relatively rare and is usually caused by lesions of the central nervous system. Gonadotropin-producing tumors, which are very rare, may cause true precocious puberty in both sexes.

452. The answer is A. *(Williams, ed 6. pp 267–276. Hung, pp 232–233.)* Although the administration of exogenous adrenocorticotropic hormone or of glucocorticoids is the most common cause of Cushing's syndrome, it may also be caused by bilateral adrenal hyperplasia. In the latter case the concentration of adrenocorticotropic hormone may be normal or high. The basic abnormality, however, is thought to be in the hypothalamic-pituitary axis, not the adrenal gland, because a distinct pituitary adenoma is found in some patients. Furthermore, many patients who have undergone bilateral adrenalectomy develop Nelson's syndrome (invasive pituitary adenoma) despite receiving adequate cortisol replacement.

453. The answer is B. *(Federman, p 58. Williams, ed 6. pp 473–476. Hung, p 340.)* True hermaphrodites by definition have both ovarian and testicular tissue. Although the majority are XX (chromatin-positive), chromosomal mosaicism has been assumed to be present in all. Although their external genitalia are ambiguous, the majority of reported hermaphroditic children have been raised as males. Ductal differentiation (development of the epididymis and vas deferens or of the fallopian tubes) is dependent on the ipsilateral presence or absence of testicular tissue, which is capable of producing androgens and mullerian inhibiting factor. Uteri are usually present. Although a familial, autosomal recessive form of true hermaphroditism has been reported, the disorder usually appears sporadically; parental sex-chromosome aberrations have no known role in its pathogenesis.

454. The answer is C. *(Rudolph, ed 17. pp 1523–1528.)* Congenital hypothyroidism may be caused by an abnormality in the thyroid gland itself (primary), in the pituitary gland (secondary), or at the level of the hypothalamus (tertiary). Thus, such a newborn is expected to have low levels of T_4 and T_3 resin uptake but, depending on the site of the defect, may have low, normal, or high concentrations of TSH. The abnormalities of thyroid binding globulin would give rise to abnormal thyroid function tests but not to hypothyroidism. Newborns with congenital hypothyroidism are often clinically normal at birth and diagnosis has often been delayed for several months. Mass screening has been employed to diagnose these patients within a few weeks of life before clinical signs and symptoms become manifest in order to prevent damage to the central nervous system and mental retardation.

455. The answer is E. *(DeGroot, ed 4. p 737. Hung, pp 150–155.)* A "cold" thyroid nodule may be a benign or malignant lesion; and with the exception of anaplastic carcinomas, most thyroid malignancies are slow-growing. The management of individuals who have a "cold" nodule is controversial. A common approach is to attempt to suppress the nodule with a short course of thyroid hormone administration. If the nodule persists after three to six months, surgical excision is performed. A dysgenetic thyroid gland may appear as a neck mass; as a rule, however, it is functional and thus does not appear as a "cold" nodule on thyroid scan.

456. The answer is D. *(Williams, ed 6. pp 285–290.)* 21-Hydroxylase deficiency is the most common form of congenital adrenal hyperplasia. These patients may have an impairment of the synthesis of both cortisol and aldosterone (salt-losing form) or of cortisol alone. Infants with the severe form of the disease may present with chemical finding of hypoaldosteronism (hyponatremia and hyperkalemia). Decreased concentrations of cortisol in these patients lead to high levels of ACTH and thus hyperpigmentation of the skin and increased synthesis of adrenal androgens. Thus, female infants with 21-hydroxylase deficiency may be virilized (female pseudohermaphroditism) but males have normal external genitalia.

457. The answer is E. *(Williams, ed 6. pp 993–996.)* Patients with pseudohypoparathyroidism have the chemical findings of hypoparathyroidism (low calcium, high phosphorus) but parathyroid hormone levels are high, indicating resistance to the action of this hormone. Thus, parathyroid hormone infusion does not produce a phosphaturic response. Phenotypically, these patients have mental retardation, shortness of stature, and obesity.

458. The answer is B. *(Williams, ed 6. p 826. Hung, p 385.)* Glucose is nonenzymatically attached to hemoglobin to form glycosylated hemoglobin. The major component of this reaction proceeds very slowly and is irreversible until the hemoglobin is destroyed. The concentration of glycosylated hemoglobin thus reflects glucose concentration over the half-life of the red cell, or about two months. Two other hemoglobins (hemoglobin A1A, and A1B) have similar properties and are often measured with hemoglobin A1C.

459. The answer is D. *(Senior, Clin Perinatology 3:79, 1976. Stanbury, ed 5. p 123–124.)* Clinitest tablets react with all reducing substances whereas Clinistix (glucose oxidase) is specific for glucose. A positive reaction with the former and a negative reaction with the latter suggest the presence of a reducing substance other than glucose in the urine. Children who have hereditary fructose intolerance as well as those who have essential fructosuria have reducing substances in their urine. Fructose intolerance, which presents during infancy, causes vomiting, hypoglycemia, and jaundice. Essential (benign) fructosuria (absence of fructokinase) is a rare autosomal recessive disorder that causes no symptoms and requires no therapy.

460. The answer is B. *(Gardner, ed 2. p 482. Hung, p 217.)* Salt-losing congenital adrenal hyperplasia (adrenogenital syndrome; 21-hydroxylase deficiency) usually manifests during the first seven to ten days of life as anorexia, vomiting, diarrhea, and dehydration. Hypoglycemia also may occur. Affected infants may have increased pigmentation, and female infants show evidence of virilization — that is, ambiguous external genitalia. Hyponatremia, hyperkalemia, and urinary sodium wasting are the usual laboratory findings. Death may occur if the diagnosis is missed and appropriate treatment is not instituted. Although adrenal aplasia, an extremely rare disorder, presents a similar clinical picture, it has an earlier onset than adrenal hyperplasia, and virilization does not occur.

461. The answer is A. *(Scriver, pp 352–353. Rudolph, ed 17. p 263.)* The infant described in the question has alcaptonuria, an autosomal recessive disorder caused by a deficiency of homogentisic acid oxidase. The diagnosis is made in infants when their urine turns black on exposure to air due to the oxidation of homogentisic acid. Affected individuals are asymptomatic in childhood. In adults, ochronosis — the deposition of a bluish pigment in cartilage and fibrous tissue — develops; symptoms of arthritis may appear later. No specific treatment is available for individuals who have alcaptonuria. The other deficiencies listed in the question are found in phenylketonuria, histidinemia, maple syrup urine disease, and isovaleric acidemia, respectively.

462. The answer is B. *(Williams, ed 6. p 1127.)* Because males have only one X chromosome (and are therefore hemizygous), they are affected by recessive traits linked to that chromosome. In each cell of heterozygous females, on the other hand, one X chromosome, either the normal X or the one carrying the abnormal allele, undergoes random inactivation (Lyon hypothesis); an X-linked recessive trait thus would be only partially expressed. For example, the X-linked recessive disorder nephrogenic diabetes insipidus produces a full-blown syndrome in males but only mild polyuria and polydipsia in heterozygous females.

463. The answer is D. *(Gardner, ed 2. p 854. Harrison, p 142.)* Nutritional rickets is caused by a dietary deficiency of vitamin D and lack of exposure to sunlight. Intestinal absorption of calcium and phosphorus is diminished in vitamin D deficiency. Transient hypocalcemia stimulates the secretion of parathormone and the mobilization of calcium and phosphorus from bone; enhanced parathormone activity leads to phosphaturia and diminished excretion of calcium. In children with nutritional rickets, serum calcium concentration usually is normal and the phosphate level low. Aminoaciduria and increased serum alkaline phosphatase activity are common findings. The excretion of calcium in the urine is increased only after therapy with vitamin D has been instituted.

464. The answer is D. *(Smith, ed 3. pp 62, 64, 122, 350, 354.)* Marfan's syndrome is a genetic disorder transmitted as an autosomal dominant trait with variable expression. Individuals with this disorder usually have tall stature, arachnodactyly, subluxation of the lens, dilatation of the aorta, and dissecting aneurysm. Mental retardation is not a part of this syndrome. Vascular complications are the usual cause of death. Patients with any of the other syndromes listed have tall stature and varying degrees of mental retardation among their clinical findings.

465. The answer is D. *(Williams, ed 6. p 1139.)* Patients with testicular feminization are genotypic males with normal testes and male internal genitalia. Complete resistance to androgens causes failure of masculinization of the external genitalia, which remain female. At puberty these individuals develop normal female breasts and body habitus despite the presence of intraabdominal testes and high concentrations of testosterone. Because of resistance to androgens, these patients have scant secondary sexual hair and thus do not develop hirsutism. The other disorders listed represent syndromes of excess androgens and, therefore, may cause hirsutism.

466. The answer is D. *(Scriver, p 267.)* Maple syrup urine disease (classical branched-chain ketoaciduria) is an autosomal recessive disorder of amino acid metabolism in which the oxidative decarboxylation of branched-chain ketoacids is blocked. Because urine odor and body odor of affected individuals resemble the smell of maple syrup, the diagnosis may be suspected. The gene frequency of this disorder is approximately 1 in 250; thus, the likelihood of a union between two heterozygotes is 1 in 62,500. Because this disorder is inherited as a recessive trait, there is a 1 in 4 chance of heterozygous parents producing a homozygous offspring. Thus, the expected incidence of the disease is 1 in 250,000.

467. The answer is A. *(Cornblath, ed 2. p 191.)* Glycogen and fat stores are diminished in premature and small-for-gestational-age infants. Energy stores are inadequate to meet the energy demands after the maternal supply of glucose is interrupted at birth, and hypoglycemia ensues. Deficiency of cortisol or growth hormone is a rare cause of neonatal hypoglycemia. Insulin excess, common in infants of diabetic mothers, is unusual in other infants. Hypoglycemia associated with a deficiency of glucagon has not been well documented.

468. The answer is A. *(Rudolph, ed 17. pp 348–350. Stanburg, ed 5. pp 1255–1260.)* Wilson's disease is an autosomal recessive disorder characterized by liver disease, neurological and behavioral disturbances, renal tubular dysfunction, and eye findings. Its multisystem manifestations are caused by the deposition of copper in various tissues and therapy is aimed at the prevention of copper accumulation. The basic defect is still not known.

469. The answer is B. *(Gardner, ed 2. p 377. Root, J Pediatr 88:1, 177, 1976. Hung, pp 188–189.)* Hypocalcemia of newborn infants may be divided into two groups: early (during the first 72 hours of life) and late (after 72 hours). The most common type of early neonatal hypocalcemia is the so-called idiopathic hypocalcemia. Current data suggest that in this heterogeneous group transient hypoparathyroidism may be present; maternal hyperparathyroidism is a rare cause of transient neonatal hypoparathyroidism. Maternal complications, including diabetes mellitus and toxemia, and neonatal disorders, such as hypoxia, prematurity, sepsis, and neonatal parathyroid disease, also may cause early hypocalcemia. Hypomagnesemia and high phosphate intake are the most common factors associated with late hypocalcemia.

470. The answer is A (1, 2, 3). *(Rudolph, ed 17. pp 1205–1206.)* Patients with Bartter's syndrome often present with failure to thrive, constipation, polyuria, vomiting, and weakness. The underlying defect is probably the failure of chloride reabsorption in the ascending limb of the loop of Henle. Laboratory findings include hypokalemia, metabolic alkalosis, hyperaldosteronism, and hyperreninemia. Hypertension is not a feature of Bartter's syndrome. Patients with chronic chloride depletion (for example, low chloride diets, chronic diuretic or laxative abuse, or chloride-losing diarrhea) may present with features of Bartter's syndrome. This syndrome may be inherited as an autosomal recessive disorder.

471. The answer is B (1, 3). *(DeLuca, Annu Rev Biochem 45:631, 1976. Hung, pp 185–187.)* Ergocalciferol (vitamin D_2) and cholecalciferol (vitamin D_3) are hydroxylated in hepatic mitochondria to form 25-hydroxy vitamin D. The rate of conversion is controlled by the concentration of 25-hydroxy vitamin D. A second hydroxylation takes place in the kidney, forming either the metabolically active compound 1,25-dihydroxy vitamin D or inactive 24,25-dihydroxy vitamin D. Formation of 1,25-dihydroxy vitamin D, the rate-limiting step in the metabolism of the vitamin, is enhanced by parathormone and low plasma phosphorus levels and is inhibited by high concentrations of calcium and phosphorus. The active form of vitamin D promotes calcium absorption in the small intestine and promotes calcium resorption from bone.

472. The answer is C (2, 4). *(Gardner, ed 2. p 565. Hung, pp 284–285. Rudolph, ed 17. pp 1544–1548.)* Patients with testicular feminization, a genetic disorder transmitted as an X-linked recessive trait, are genetic males (karyotype 46,XY) with normal female external genitalia. The syndrome is caused by peripheral androgen resistance due to an abnormality of receptors within the cytosol; as a result, androgen translocation into the nucleus, a crucial step in mediating androgen action, fails to occur. Diagnosis is made either during infancy or childhood when testicular tissue is found in a hernial sac at herniorrhaphy or after puberty when affected individuals present with primary amenorrhea. Well-developed vasa deferentia and epididymes are usually present; and although there is no uterus, rudimentary mullerian elements may be discovered. At puberty, individuals with testicular feminization undergo normal female breast development and may grow small amounts of sexual hair.

473. The answer is A (1, 2, 3). *(DeGroot, pp 1451–1454.)* Most hirsute women have no demonstrable endocrine disorder. A genetic or constitutional cause is usually the basis for hairiness in women; for instance, Orientals and American Indians have scant body hair, whereas dark-haired individuals from Middle Eastern and Mediterranean countries tend to be hirsute. Development of sexual hair in females is dependent on the low concentration of androgens from the adrenal glands and ovaries. Excess androgen production by these organs is responsible for hirsutism in a minority of cases. Testicular tissue is not present in women. If it is present, the individual is, by definition, a hermaphrodite and usually presents with ambiguous genitalia.

474. The answer is E (all). *(Williams, ed 6. pp 180, 212, 382–390.)* Hypogonadotropic hypogonadism caused by either hypothalamic or pituitary failure leads to ovarian understimulation and primary or secondary amenorrhea. Ovarian function is also influenced by other endocrine disorders. Hyperprolactinemia is a common cause of secondary amenorrhea and may also cause primary amenorrhea. Abnormalities of the thyroid gland (both hypo- and hyperthyroidism) also are among causes of the disturbances of ovarian function and amenorrhea.

475. The answer is A. (1, 2, 3). *(Senior, Pediatr Clin N Am 26:171, 1979. Hung, pp 375–376.)* In the immediate postabsorptive state, glycogen stores are metabolized to meet energy requirements. In fasting, however, as the supply of glycogen diminishes, the body must gradually switch to lipid metabolism. Accordingly, insulin concentration is diminished and lipolysis and ketogenesis are enhanced. Serum free fatty acids and ketones are at high levels and are used as fuel. Glucose utilization diminishes and glucose concentration is maintained at a level commensurate with the ability of the body to use alternate fuels.

476. The answer is A (1, 2, 3). *(DeGroot, p 1826. Williams, ed 6. p 618. Hung, pp 64–66.)* The concentration of human growth hormone in blood varies markedly but with no regular periodicity in the course of 24 hours. There is a surge of growth hormone secretion during deep sleep (stage IV); lower values are associated with the rapid eye movement stage of sleep. Growth hormone concentrations can be increased by various stimuli including hypoglycemia, stress, and exercise. Certain amino acids (primarily arginine), vasopressin, pyrogen, and L-dopa can also increase growth hormone levels. Although their mode of action is unknown, these stimuli can be used to distinguish normal children from those who are growth-hormone-deficient because the latter will not exhibit increases in growth hormone levels. Medroxyprogesterone acetate has not been used as a stimulus for growth hormone secretion.

477. The answer is E (all). *(Gardner, ed 2. p 103. Hung, p 81.)* Tall stature in children usually is familial and cannot be traced to an underlying physiologic or metabolic abnormality. Causes of nonfamilial tall stature include pituitary gigantism (growth hormone excess), cerebral gigantism, Marfan's syndrome, homocystinuria, and chromosomal disorders, including karyotypes 47,XXY (Klinefelter's syndrome) and 47,XYY. Patients with congenital adrenal hyperplasia are tall as children but become short adults. Although boys rarely complain of tall stature, excessive height may pose psychosocial problems for girls. The use of estrogens to accelerate epiphyseal closure and reduce final adult height in girls has been advocated in the past. However, in view of the possible carcinogenicity of estrogens, this therapy must be used with caution.

478. The answer is A (1, 2, 3). *(Rudolph, ed 17. pp 267–268.)* Patients with hyperlacticacidemia are a heterogeneous group with various inherited enzymatic defects. Biochemically, they are characterized by acidosis and elevated concentrations of lactate. A defect in the metabolism of pyruvate is often the underlying abnormality. Fasting hypoglycemia may be present. Patients with a deficiency of a gluconeogenic enzyme (pyruvate carboxyglase, phosphoenolpyruvate carboxy-kinase, and fructose-1, 6-diphosphatase) and those with a deficiency of pyruvate dehydrogenase complex may have hyperlacticacidemia. Phosphofructokinase is an enzyme of the glycolytic pathyway and its deficiency will not give rise to high lactate levels.

479. The answer is A (1, 2, 3). *(Gardner, ed 2. p 226. Hung, pp 128, 134)* Infants with congenital hypothyroidism may not manifest any symptoms or signs in the early weeks of life. Patients with secondary or tertiary hypothyroidism will have a normal (lower limit of the assay) concentration of thyroid-stimulating hormone and low levels of thyroxine. Most of the thyroid hormone in the circulation is protein bound, predominantly to thyroxine-binding globulin and thyroxine-binding prealbumin. Only the unbound (free) fraction is metabolically active; it regulates the pituitary secretion of thyroid-stimulating hormone by a negative feedback mechanism. In thyroxine-binding globulin deficiency, a hereditary disorder transmitted as an X-linked dominant trait, total thyroxine concentration is low although free thyroxine concentration is normal. Individuals who have this disorder have a normal metabolic rate and normal serum concentration of thyroid-stimulating hormone. This infant does not have primary hypothyroidism, in which one would expect a low level of thyroxine and a high concentration of thyroid-stimulating hormone.

480. The answer is A (1, 2, 3). *(Federman, p 143. Rudolph, ed 17. pp 1542–1545. Gardner, ed 2. pp 476, 500, 571.)* The most common cause of ambiguous genitalia in female infants is congenital adrenal hyperplasia (21-hydroxylase deficiency). Maternal ingestion of androgens or progestins, the latter usually prescribed because of a threatened abortion, also may virilize a female fetus. True hermaphroditism, which is due to the presence of both ovarian and testicular tissue in the same individual, is a rare cause. Infants who have neonatal Cushing's syndrome present with massive obesity, plethora, and thinning of the skin but no evidence of virilization.

481. The answer is B (1, 3). *(Stanbury, ed 5 p 231. Williams, ed 6. pp 219–222.)* In the presence of a normal pituitary gland, a deficiency of thyroid hormones causes an elevation in thyroid-stimulating hormone levels and enlargement of the thyroid gland. Five familial disorders of thyroid hormone synthesis, including peroxidase deficiency, iodide transport defect, failure of iodotyrosine coupling, failure of iodotyrosine deiodinase activity, and altered thyroglobulin synthesis, cause goiter and hypothyroidism in neonates. In addition, maternal ingestion of goitrogens (e.g., iodide or antithyroid drugs), which cross the placenta, may cause neonatal hypothyroidism. Deficiency of thyroid-stimulating hormone may produce neonatal hypothyroidism but not gland enlargement. Thyroid hormone does not cross the placenta, and therefore, maternal ingestion would be neither beneficial nor harmful to a fetus.

482. The answer is B (1, 3). *(Gardner, ed 2. p 138. Rudolph, ed 17. p 297, 1162, 1476.)* Children with diabetes mellitus in early stages classically present with polyuria, polydipsia, and polyphagia. Later on, anorexia rather than polyphagia is a frequent complaint. Central diabetes insipidus is caused by a deficiency of vasopressin (antidiuretic hormone). Because the renal collecting tubules are impermeable to water, hypotonic urine is formed. Polyuria, thirst, polydipsia, and anorexia are characteristic. Children with nephrogenic diabetes insipidus have similar findings but become symptomatic shortly after birth. Phosphate diabetes (hypophosphatemic rickets) presents with the characteristic signs and symptoms of rickets and not with polyuria and polydipsia.

483–487. The answers are: 483-A, 484-E, 485-D, 486-B, 487-D. *(Harrison, pp 84, 117, 219, 258. Williams, ed 6. p 232.)* Vitamin D-resistant rickets is caused by a genetic abnormality in the renal tubular absorption of phosphate with resultant hyperphosphaturia and hypophosphatemia. No other renal tubular abnormality is present. The intestinal absorption of phosphate is also abnormal and calcium absorption from the gut may be secondarily affected. Calcium concentration is usually normal. The disorder is transmitted as an X-linked dominant trait.

Patients with pseudohypoparathyroidism have the same chemical abnormality (low Ca, high PO_4) as those with hypoparathyroidism. They are distinguished from the latter group by their phenotypic features and high serum concentration of parathormone. The basic abnormality in these patients is the unresponsiveness of the renal tubules to parathyroid hormone. They are classified into two groups depending on the site of the defect. Type I patients have failure to generate cyclic AMP and do not have an increase in urinary concentration of cyclic AMP or phosphate in response to parathyroid hormone. Type II patients have a defect in the renal tubules which causes failure to respond to high concentrations of cyclic AMP. These patients, if given parathyroid hormone, have increased urinary excretion of cyclic AMP but not of phosphate.

Osteogenesis imperfecta is a genetic disorder transmitted as an autosomal recessive (severe form) or, more commonly, autosomal dominant (mild form) trait. The basic defect is an abnormality in the production and composition of the matrix of bone cells. Serum calcium and phosphate concentrations are normal.

Hyperparathyroidism is rare in children. In response to high concentrations of parathyroid hormone there is increased bone resorption. In the kidney there is increased excretion of phosphate and enhanced formation of 1,25-dihydroxy vitamin D. Increased formation of 1,25-dihydroxy vitamin D in turn enhances the absorption of calcium and, secondarily, of phosphorus from the gut. The net effect is hypercalcemia and hypophosphatemia.

Medullary carcinoma of thyroid arises from the C cells of the thyroid. These tumors secrete excessive amounts of calcitonin and accordingly the concentration of this hormone in the blood is increased. Despite elevated levels of calcitonin, the serum concentration of calcium and of phosphorus is usually normal unless the patient has associated hyperparathyroidism (multiple endocrine adenomatosis, type II).

488–493. The answers are: 488-E, 489-A, 490-B, 491-E, 492-E, 493-B. *(Gardner, ed 2. pp 500, 1324, 1333. Wilkins, ed 3. p 262. Williams, ed 6. pp 267–270. Smith, ed 3. pp 152, 324, 442.)* The Prader-Willi syndrome is a disorder consisting of hypotonia, hypogonadism, hyperphagia, and varying degrees of mental retardation. Children affected by this syndrome exhibit little movement in utero and are hypotonic during the neonatal period. Feeding difficulties and failure to thrive may be the presenting complaints in the first year; later, obesity becomes the most common presenting complaint. The enormous food intake of affected children is thought to be due to a defect in the satiety center in the hypothalamus. Stringent caloric restriction is the only known treatment.

Laurence-Moon-Biedl syndrome is transmitted as an autosomal recessive trait. Obesity, mental retardation, hypogonadism, polydactyly, and retinitis pigmentosa with night blindness are the principal findings in affected children. There is no known effective treatment.

The initial complaint in Cushing's syndrome may be obesity. Accumulation of fat in the face, neck, and trunk causes the characteristic "buffalo hump" and "moon" facies. Characteristic features include growth failure, muscle wasting, thinning of the skin, plethora, and hypertension. The bone age of affected patients is retarded, and osteoporosis may be present. The disorder results from an excess of glucocorticoids that may be caused by a primary adrenal abnormality (adenoma or carcinoma) or secondary hypercortisolism, which may be due to excess adrenocorticotropin. Exogenous glucocorticoids administered in supraphysiologic doses for a prolonged period of time will produce a similar picture in normal subjects.

Pseudohypoparathyroidism is a familial disorder transmitted as an X-linked trait. Affected patients have biochemical findings (low serum calcium and high serum phosphorus levels) similar to those associated with hypoparathyroidism, but they also have high levels of endogenous parathormone; in addition, exogenous parathormone fails to increase their phosphate excretion or raise their serum calcium level. The defect in these patients appears to be either at the hormone receptor site or in the adenylate cyclase-cyclic AMP system. The symptoms of pseudohypoparathyroidism are due to hypocalcemia. Affected children are short, round-faced, and mildly retarded. Metacarpals and metatarsals are shortened, and metastatic calcifications, basal ganglia calcifications, and cataracts may be present. The current treatment consists of large doses of vitamin D and reduction of the phosphate load.

Frohlich's syndrome was described originally in an obese boy with sexual infantilism and shortness of stature but is no longer used as a diagnostic term.

494–500. The answers are: 494-A, 495-E, 496-E, 497-D, 498-B, 499-A, 500-B. *(Gardner, ed 2. pp 138, 145, 478, 511. Hung, pp 105, 109, 110, 227, 240.)* In the salt-losing variety of 21-hydroxylase deficiency, the synthesis of both mineralocorticoids (e.g., aldosterone) and cortisol is impaired. Aldosterone deficiency impairs the exchange of potassium for sodium in the distal renal tubule. Affected patients have hyponatremia and hyperkalemia. Dehydration, hypotension, and shock may be present.

In the absence of vasopressin, renal collecting tubules are impermeable to water, resulting in the excretion of hypotonic urine. Patients with diabetes insipidus present with polyuria and polydipsia. Net loss of water leads to dehydration and hemoconcentration and, therefore, to relatively high serum concentrations of sodium and potassium. Patients with nephrogenic diabetes insipidus have similar laboratory findings. This genetic disorder is unresponsive to antidiuretic hormone (ADH). These patients are unable to concentrate their urine and present in the neonatal period with hypernatremic dehydration.

In hyperaldosteronism, renal tubular sodium-potassium exchange is enhanced. Hypokalemia, hypernatremia, hyperchloremia, and akalosis are the usual findings. Primary hyperaldosteronism (Conn's syndrome) is very rare in children.

The hallmark of the syndrome of inappropriate secretion of antidiuretic hormone is the coexistence of hyponatremia, overhydration, and inappropriately high concentrations of sodium in the urine. Levels of serum potassium that are slightly lower than normal are the consequence of dilution and secondary hyperaldosteronism.

Addison's disease is associated with a combined deficiency of glucocorticoids and mineralocorticoids. Resorption of sodium and excretion of potassium and hydrogen ions are impaired at the level of the distal renal tubules. Sodium loss results in loss of water and depletion of blood volume. Individuals with compensated Addison's disease may have relatively normal physical and laboratory findings; Addisonian crisis, however, characteristically produces hyponatremia, hyperkalemia, and shock. The pathophysiology of the serum electrolyte abnormalities in this disorder is the same as in the salt-losing variety of adrenogenital syndrome.

Patients with a deficiency of glucose-6-phosphatase (von Gierke's disease) are, as a rule, hyperlipemic. Increased triglyceride concentration in the serum decreases the volume and solute content of the aqueous compartment. Because electrolytes are present only in the aqueous compartment of the serum but are expressed in milliequivalents per liter of serum as a whole, the concentrations of sodium and potassium are factitiously low in these patients.

Bibliography

Adams F, Emmanouilides G (eds): *Moss' Heart Disease in Infants, Children and Adolescents,* 3rd ed. Baltimore, Waverly Press, 1983.

Adams RA, Lyons G: *Neurology of Hereditary Metabolic Diseases of Children.* New York, McGraw-Hill, 1982.

Alpert E: Pathogenesis of arthritis associated with viral hepatitis. *N Engl J Med* 285:185–189, 1971.

Altman AJ, Schwartz AD: *Malignant Diseases of Infancy, Childhood and Adolescence,* 2nd ed. Philadelphia, WB Saunders, 1983.

American Academy of Pediatrics, American College of Obstetrics and Gynecology: *Guidelines for Perinatal Care,* 1983.

American Academy of Pediatrics, Committee on Nutrition: Iron supplementation for infants. *Pediatrics* 58:765, 1976.

Anderson RH, McCartney FJ, Shinebourne EA: *Pediatric Cardiology,* vol 5., 1983

Avery GB (ed): *Neonatology: Pathophysiology and Management of the Newborn,* 2nd ed. Philadephpia, JB Lippincott, 1981.

Avery ME, Taeusch GR Jr (eds): *Schaffer's Diseases of the Newborn,* 5th ed. Philadelphia, WB Saunders, 1984.

Baraff LJ, Wilkins J, Wehrle PF: The role of antibiotics, immunization, and adenoviruses in pertussis. *Pediatrics* 61:224–230, 1978.

Behrman RE, Vaughan VC III, Nelson WE: *Nelson Textbook of Pediatrics,* 12th ed. Philadelphia, WB Saunders, 1983.

Bell WE, McCormick WF: *Increased Intracranial Pressure in Children,* 2nd ed., vol 8. Philadelphia, WB Saunders, 1978.

Bell WE, McCormick WF: *Neurologic Infections in Children,* vol 12. Philadephia, WB Saunders, 1978.

Bergman I, et al: Neonatal seizures. *Semin Perinatol* 6:54–67, 1982.

Black PM: Brain death. *N Engl J Med* 299:338–344, 1978.

Blacklow NR: Viral gastroenteritis. *N Engl J Med* 304:397–406, 1981.

Bowman JM: *Current Problems in Pediatric Hematology.* New York: Grune & Stratton, 1975.

Braunwald E: *Heart Disease: A Textbook of Cardiovascular Medicine,* 2nd ed. Philadelphia, WB Saunders, 1984.

Brooke MH: *A Clinician's View of Neuromuscular Diseases.* Baltimore, Williams & Wilkins, 1977.

Brown JK: Migraine and migraine equivalents in children. *Develop Med Child Neurol* 19:683–692, 1977.

Browne TB: Valproic acid. *N Engl J Med* 302:661–665, 1980.

Caffey J, et al: *Pediatric X-Ray Diagnosis,* 7th ed. Chicago, Year Book Medical, 1978.

Cines DB, Dusak B, Tomaski A, et al: Immune thromboytopenia and pregnancy. *N Engl J Med* 306:826, 1982.

Congdon PJ, Forsythe WI: Migraine in childhood: a study of 300 children. *Develop Med Child Neurol* 21:209–216, 1979.

Cornblath M, Schwartz R: *Disorders of Carbohydrate Metabolism in Infancy,* 2nd ed. Philadelphia, WB Saunders, 1976.

Dallman PR: Iron deficiency in infancy and childhood. *Report of the International Nutritional Anemia Consultative Group (INACG),* 1979.

D'Angio GJ: Wilms' tumor: an update. *Cancer* 45:1791–1798, 1980.

D'Angio GJ, Evans A, Breslaw N, Beckwith B, et al: The treatment of Wilms' tumor: results of the Second National Wilms' Tumor Study. *Cancer* 47(9):2302–2311, 1981.

DeGroot LJ (ed): *Endocrinology.* New York, Grune & Stratton, 1979.

DeGroot LJ, Stanbury JB: *The Thyroid Diseases,* 4th ed. New York, John Wiley, 1975.

Delgado-Escueta AV, et al: *Advances in Neurology,* New York, Raven Press, 1983.

De Luca HF, Schnoes HK: Metabolism and mechanism of action of vitamin D. *Annu Rev Biochem* 45:631, 1976.

Denny FW, Clyde WA Jr, Gelzen WP: Mycoplasma pneumoniae disease: clinical spectrum, pathophysiology, epidemiology, and control. *J Infect Dis* 123:74, 1971.

DeVivo DC, Keating, JP, Haymond MW: Acute encephalopathy with fatty infiltration of the viscera. *Pediatr Clin North Am* 23:527–540, 1976.

Dillon HC: Impetigo contagiosa: suppurative and non-suppurative complications. *Am J Dis Child* 115:530–541, 1968.

Dodge PR: Myotonic dystrophy in infancy and childhood. *Pediatrics* 35:3–19, 1965.

Dodge PR, Swartz MN: Bacterial meningitis–a review of selected aspects. *N Engl J Med* 272:954–960, 1003–1010, 1965.

Dubowitz V: *Muscle Disorders in Childhood*, vol 16. Philadelphia, WB Saunders, 1978.

Faerø O, Kastrup KW, Nielson EL, et al: Successful prophylaxis of febrile convulsions with phenobarbital. *Epilepsia* 13:279–285, 1972.

Fanaroff AA, Martin RJ (eds): *Behrman's Neonatal Perinatal Medicine,* 3rd ed. St. Louis, CV Mosby, 1983.

Feder HM Jr: Occult pneumococcal bacteremia and the febrile infant and young child–clinical review. *Clin Pediatr* 19:457–462, 1980.

Federman DD: *Abnormal Sexual Development.* Philadelphia, WB Saunders, 1967.

Fekety R: Recent advances in bacterial diarrhea. *Rev Infect Dis* 5:246–257, 1983.

Feldman WE: Effect of ampicillin and chlormaphenicol against Hemophilus influenzae. *Pediatrics* 61:406–409, 1978.

Fishman RA: *Cerebrospinal Fluid in Diseases of the Nervous System.* Philadelphia, WB Saunders, 1980.

Fleischer GR: Falsely normal radionucleide scans for osteomyelitis. *Am J Dis Child* 134:499–502, 1980.

Friedman WF, Lesch M, Sonnenblick EH (eds): *Neonatal Heart Disease.* New York, Grune & Stratton, 1973.

Gardner LI: *Endocrine and Genetic Diseases of Childhood and Adolescence,* 2nd ed. Philadelphia, WB Saunders, 1975.

Gellis SS (ed): *Year Book of Pediatrics.* Chicago, Year Book Medical, 1978.

Gellis SS, Kagan BM (eds): *Current Pediatric Therapy,* 11th ed. Philadelphia, WB Saunders, 1984.

Goldman P, Peppercorn MA: Drug therapy: sulfasalazine. *N Engl J Med* 293:20–23, 1975.

Gordon N: *Pediatric Neurology for the Clinician.* Philadelphia, JB Lippincott, 1976.

Greenberger N: Medium chain triglycerides, physiological considerations and clinical implications. *N Engl J Med* 280:1045–1058, 1969.

Greseon NT, Kirkpatrick JA, Gradang BR, et al: Gastric antral narrowing in chronic granulomatous disease of childhood. *Pediatrics* 54:456, 1974.

Gryboski J, Walker A: *Gastrointestinal Problems in the Infant,* 2nd ed. Philadelphia, WB Saunders, 1983.

Guggenheim MA, et al: Progressive neuromuscular disease in children with chronic cholestasis and vitamin E deficiency: diagnosis and treatment with alpha tocopherol. *J Pediatr* 100:51–58, 1982.

Halliday JW, Powell LW: Iron overload. *Semin Hematol* 19(1):42–53, 1982.

Hallman M, Gluck L: Respiratory distress syndrome – update 1982. *Pediatr-Clin North Am* 29:1057–1075, 1982.

Handsfield HH, et al: Epidemiology of penicillinase-producing Neisseria gonorrhoeae infections. *N Engl J Med* 306:950–954, 1982.

Harper PS: *Myotonic Dystrophy.* Philadelphia, WB Saunders, 1979.

Harrison HE, Harrison HC: *Disorders of Calcium and Phosphate Metabolism in Childhood and Adolescence.* Philadelphia, WB Saunders, 1979.

Higby DJ: Granulocyte transfusions: current status. *Blood* 55:2–8, 1980.

Hoekleman RA, et al (eds): *Principles of Pediatrics: Health Care of the Young.* New York, McGraw-Hill, 1978.

Hopkins CC, Dismukes WE, Glick TH, et al: Surveillance of paralytic poliomyelitis in the United States. *JAMA* 210:694–700, 1969.

Hrachovy RA, et al: Double-blind study of ACTH vs prednisone therapy in infantile spasms. *J Pediatr* 103:641–645, 1983.

Hung W, August GP, Glasgow AM: *Pediatric Endocrinology.* New Hyde Park, N.Y., Medical Examination Publishing, 1983.

Illingworth RS: *The Development of the Infant and Young Child: Abnormal and Normal,* 7th ed. New York, Longman, 1980.

Isler W: *Clinics in Developmental Medicine.* New York, JB Lippincott, 1971.

Jennett B: *Epilepsy After Non-Missile Head Injuries,* 2nd ed. Chicago, Year Book Medical, 1975.

Karayalcin G, Hassani N, Abrams M: Cholelithiasis in children with sickle cell disease. *Am J Dis Child* 233:306, 1979.

Katz SL: Ampicillin-resistant Hemophilus influenzae type b: a status report. *Pediatrics* 55:6–8, 1975.

Keith JD, Rowe RD, Vlad P: *Heart Disease in Infancy and Childhood,* 3rd ed. New York, Macmillan, 1978.

Kelly DH, Shannon DC: Periodic breathing in infants with near-miss sudden infant death syndrome. *Pediatrics* 63:355–360, 1979.

Kerr DN, Harrison CV, Sherlock S, et al: Congenital hepatic fibrosis. *Q J Med* 30:91–117, 1961.

Kliegman RM, Fanaroff AA: Necrotizing enterocolitis. *N Engl J Med* 310:1093–1103,1984

Kohl S: Yersinia enterocolitica infections in children. *Pediatr Clin North Am* 26:433–443, 1979.

Krugman S, Ward R, Katz SC: *Infectious Diseases of Children,* 7th ed. St. Louis, CV Mosby, 1980.

Lancet (editorial): Prevention of perinatally transmitted hepatitis B infection. 1:939–941, 1984.

Levine, AD (ed): *Cancer in the Young.* Masson Publishing USA, 1982.

Lindenbaum J: megaloblastic anemia and neutrophil hypersegmentation. *Br J Haematol* 44:511–513, 1979.

Lipton JM, Nathan DG: Aplastic and hypoplastic anemia. *Pediatr Clin North Am* 27:217–235, 1980.

Luban NLC, Leikin SL, August GA: Growth and development in sickle cell anemia:preliminary report. *Am J Pediatr Hematol/Oncol* 4(1):61–65, 1982.

Lumicao GG, Heggie AD: Chlamydial infections. *Pediatr Clin North Am* 26:269–282, 1979.

Lux SE, Wolfe LC: Inherited disorders of the red cell membrane skeleton. *Pediatr Clin North Am* 27:463–486, 1980.

Mauer AM: Therapy of acute lymphoblastic leukemia in childhood. *Blood* 56:1–10, 1980.

McRae DL: Observations on craniolacunia. *Acta Radiol* (Diagn) 5:55–64, 1966.

Meissner HC: Lyme disease first observed to be aseptic meningitis. *Am J Dis Child* 136:465–467, 1982.

Meissner HC, Smith AL: The current status of chloramphenicol. *Pediatrics* 64:348–356, 1979.

Menkes JH: *Textbook of Child Neurology,* 2nd ed. Philadelphia, Lea & Febiger, 1980.

Monreal FJ: Asymmetric crying facies: an alternative interpretation. *Pediatrics* 65:146–149, 1980.

Nadas AS, Fyler DC: *Pediatric Cardiology,* 3rd ed. Philadelphia, WB Saunders, 1972.

Nathan DG, Oski FA: *Hematology of Infancy and Childhood,* 2nd ed. Philadelphia, WB Saunders, 1981.

Nelson KB, Ellenberg JH: Predictors of epilepsy in children who have experienced febrile seizures. *N Engl J Med* 295:1029–1033, 1976.

Nelson KB, Eng G: Congenital hypoplasia of the depressor anguli oris muscle: differentiation from congenital facial palsy. *J Pediatr* 81: 16–20,1972.

Neville BG: Central nervous system involvement in leukemia. *Dev Med Child Neurol* 14:75–78, 1972.

Oski FA, Naiman JL: *Hematologic Problems in the Newborn,* 3rd ed. Philadelphia, WB Saunders, 1982.

ication. *Pediatr Clin North Am* 27:237–253, 1980.

Pape KE, Pickering D: Asymmetric crying facies: an index of other congenital anomalies. *J Pediatr* 81:21–30, 1972.

Partin JD: Mitchondrial ultra-structure in Reye's syndrome. *N Engl J Med* 285:1139–1143, 1971.

Perloff JK: *The Clinical Recognition of Congenital Heart Disease,* 2nd ed. Philadelphia, WB Saunders, 1978.

Peter G, Smith AL: Group A streptococcal infections of the skin and pharynx. *N Engl J Med* 297:311–317, 365–370, 1977.

Petersdorf RG, et al: *Harrison's Principles of Internal Medicine,* 10th ed. New York, McGraw-Hill, 1983.

Phelps DL: Neonatal oxygen toxicity: Is it preventable? *Pediatr Clin North Am* 29:1233–1240, 1982.

Piomelli S, Brickman A, Carlos E: Rapid diagnosis of iron deficiency by measurement of FEP/hemoglobin ration. *Pediatrics* 57:136–141, 1976.

Plum F, Posner JB: *The Diagnosis of Stupor and Coma,* 3rd ed. Philadelphia, FA Davis, 1980.

Pollack JD: *Reye's Syndrome.* New York, Grune & Stratton, 1975.

Prensky AL, Sommer D: Diagnosis and treatment of migraine in children. *Neurology* 29:506–510, 1979.

Price RA, Jamieson PA: The central nervous system in childhood leukemia. II. Subacute leucoencephalopathy. *Cancer* 35:306–318, 1975.

Prince AS, Neu HC: Antibiotic-associated pseudomembranous colitis in children. *Pediatr Clin North Am* 26:261–268, 1979.

Reye RD: Encephalopathy and fatty degeneration of the viscera: a disease entity in childhood. *Lancet* 2:749–757, 1963.

Roberts WC: *Cardiology.* New York, Yorke Medical Books, 1983.

Root AW, Harrison HE: Recent advances in calcium metabolism. *J Pediatr* 88:1–18, 177–179, 1976.

Rowland TW, et al: Brain death in the pediatric intensive care unit. *Am J Dis Child* 137:547–550, 1983.

Rubenstein L, Herman MM, Long TF, et al: Disseminated necrotizing leucoencephalopathy: a complication of treated central nervous system leukemia and lymphoma. *Cancer* 35:291–305, 1975.

Rudolph AM, et al (eds): *Pediatrics,* 17th ed. New York, Appleton-Century-Crofts, 1982.

Saarinen UM : Serum ferritin in assessment of iron nutrition in healthy infants. *Acta Paediatr Scand* 67:745, 1978.

Sabesin SM, Koff RS: Pathogenesis of experimental viral hepatitis. *N Engl J Med* 290:944–950, 996–1002, 1974.

Sanford JP: Legionnaire's disease–the first thousand days. *N Engl J Med* 300:654–656, 1979.

Sato S, et al: Valproic acid versus ethosurimide in the treatment of absence seizures. *Neurology* 32:157–163, 1982.

Schaffer AJ, Avery ME: *Diseases of the Newborn,* 4th ed. Philadelphia, WB Saunders, 1977.

Schapiro RL: *Clinical Radiology of the Pediatric Abdomen Gastrointestinal Tract.* Baltimore, University Park Press, 1979.

Scharli, A, Sieber WK, Kiesewetter WB: Hypertrophic pyloric stenosis at Children's Hospital of Pittsburgh from 1912 to 1967: a critical view. *J Pediatr Surg* 4:108–114, 1969.

Schiff L: *Diseases of the Liver,* 4th ed. Philadelphia, JB Lippincott, 1975.

Scriver CR, Rosenberg LE: *Amino Acid Metabolism and Its Disorders.* Philadelphia, WB Saunders, 1973.

Senior B, Sadeghi-Nejad A: The glycogenoses and other inherited disorders of carbohydrate metabolism. *Clin Perinatol* 3:79, 1976.

Senior B, Wolfsdorf JI: Hypoglycemia in children. *Pediatr Clin North Am* 26:171–185, 1979.

Seto DSY: Viral hepatitis. *Pediatr Clin North Am* 26:305–314, 1979.

Shapiro AK, Shapiro E: Tourette syndrome: clinical aspects, treatment, and etiology. *Semin Neurol* 2:373–385, 1982.

Silverman A, Roy CC, Cozzetto FJ: *Pediatric Clinical Gastronenterology,* 3rd ed. St. Louis, CV Mosby, 1983.

Singer WD, Rabe EF, Haller JS: The effect of ACTH therapy upon infantile spasms. *J Pediatr* 96:485–489, 1980.

Sleisenger MH, Fordtran JS: *Gastrointestinal Disease: Pathophysiology, Diagnosis, Management,* 3rd ed. Philadelphia, WB Saunders, 1983.

Smith DW: *Recognizable Patterns of Human Malformation: Genetic, Embryologic and Clinical Aspects,* 3rd ed. Philadelphia, WB Saunders, 1982.

Stanbury JB, Wyngaarden JB, Fredrickson DS: The Metabolic Basis of Inherited Disease, 5th ed. New York, McGraw-Hill, 1983.

Steinhoff MC: Rotavirus: the first five years. *J Pediatr* 96:611–622, 1980.

Sullivan DW: Hereditary spherocytosis. *Pediatr Ann* 9:38–42, 1980.

Sullivan JL: Epstein-Barr virus and X-linked lymphoproliferative syndrome *Adv Pediatr* 31:365–399, 1984.

Swaiman DF, Wright FS(eds): *The Practice of Pediatric Neurology.* 2nd ed. St. Louis, CV Mosby, 1982.

Taylor-Robinson D, McCormack WM: The genital mycoplasmas. *N Engl J Med* 302:1003–1010, 1063–1067, 1980.

Thomsett MJ, et al: Endocrine and neurologic outcome in childhood craniophary-ngioma: review of effect of treatment in 42 patients. *J Pediatr* 97:728–735, 1980.

Thompson JA: Infant botulism: clinical spectrum and epidemiology. *Pediatrics* 66:936–942, 180.

Tipple, MA, Been NO, Saxon EM: Clinial characteristics of the afebrile pneumonia associated with *Chlamydia trachomatis* infection in infants less than 6 months of age. *Pediatrics* 63:192–197, 1979.

Torphy DD, Bond WW: *Campylobacter* fetus infections in children. *Pediatrics* 64:896–903, 1979.

Trier JS: Diagnostic value per oral biopsy of the proximal small intestine. *N Engl J Med* 285:1470, 1973.

Volpe, JJ: *Neurology of the Newborn.* Philadelphia, W.B. Saunders, 1981.

Walton JN: *Disorders of Voluntary Muscle,* 4th ed. New York, Churchill-Livingston, 1981.

Watson H (ed): *Pediatric Cardiology.* St. Louis, CV Mosby, 1968.

Westmoreland BF: *Tuberous Sclerosis,* M Gomez (ed). New York, Raven Press, 1979.

Wilkins L: *The Diagnosis and Treatment of Endocrine Disorders in Childhood and Adolescence,* 3rd ed. Springfield, CC Thomas, 1966.

Williams RH (ed): *Textbook of Endocrinology,* 6th ed. Philadelphia, WB Saunders, 1981.

Williams WJ, et al: *Hematology,* 2nd ed. New York, McGraw-Hill, 1977.

Yow MD, Katz SL: *Red Book,* 18th ed. Evanston, Illinois, American Academy of Pediatrics, Report of the Committee on Infectious Diseases, 1977.

Zieve, L: Pathogenesis of hepatic coma. *Arch Intern Med* 118:211–223, 1966.